MW01657105

Fenbendazole & Ivermectin Protocols

A Practical Handbook for Cancer Patients and Caregivers, with Research-Based Treatment, Patient Experiences, and Step-by-Step Checklists

Andrew Kerrington

Disclaimer

This book is intended for **educational and informational purposes only**. It summarizes published research and patient-reported experiences regarding the non-traditional use of certain medications in cancer contexts.

- It is **not** intended to provide medical advice, diagnosis, or treatment.
- It does **not** recommend or endorse any specific therapy, dosage, or regimen.
- Always seek the advice of a qualified physician or other licensed healthcare provider with any questions regarding a medical condition or before starting, stopping, or changing any medication or treatment plan.
- Off-label use of prescription or veterinary drugs may involve significant health risks, potential drug interactions, and legal or regulatory considerations.

The author and publisher disclaim any liability for any loss, injury, or damage allegedly arising from the use or misuse of the information contained herein. Reliance on any information provided in this book is **solely at your own risk**.

Table of Content

PART I
GETTING STARTED

CHAPTER 1: WELCOME & IMPORTANT NOTES

1.1 A PERSONAL WELCOME TO PATIENTS AND CAREGIVERS

Every journey through cancer is deeply personal, shaped by moments of uncertainty, hope, and the relentless search for clarity. Whether you are facing a diagnosis yourself or standing beside someone you care for, you have already demonstrated a remarkable commitment to understanding and navigating the complexities of cancer care. This book was written with that commitment in mind, drawing on both scientific rigor and the lived experiences of patients and caregivers who have walked this path before you.

In recent years, the conversation around *integrative approaches* to cancer treatment has grown more nuanced. Patients and their loved ones are increasingly seeking information about therapies that exist outside the boundaries of conventional protocols. Among these, fenbendazole and ivermectin have emerged as topics of significant interest and debate. The information available online is often fragmented, sometimes contradictory, and rarely tailored to the practical realities faced by those living with cancer. Recognizing this gap, the intent here is to provide a resource that is both authoritative and accessible—a guide that empowers you to make informed decisions in collaboration with your healthcare team.

What distinguishes this handbook is its foundation in *evidence-based research* combined with the voices of those who have firsthand experience. The protocols discussed are not presented as miracle cures or substitutes for established medical care. Instead, they are explored with the same critical lens that guides responsible medical inquiry. Throughout these pages, you will find clear explanations of scientific studies, practical checklists to help you organize and monitor your approach, and candid accounts from individuals who have chosen to integrate these agents into their care. The aim is not to offer false hope, but rather to foster a sense of agency and partnership in your care decisions.

Navigating cancer is rarely straightforward. The sheer volume of information, the rapid pace of new research, and the emotional weight of each decision can be overwhelming. In compiling this book, every effort has been made to distill complex concepts into language that is precise, yet approachable. Where uncertainty exists in the literature, it is acknowledged openly. Where patient experiences diverge, those differences are explored thoughtfully, providing a spectrum of perspectives rather than a single narrative. This approach is grounded in respect for your intelligence and your right to understand the full context of any treatment option you may consider.

The practical tools included—step-by-step planning guides, concise reference charts, and communication strategies for engaging with your medical team—are designed to reduce confusion and help you track your progress. These resources are not a substitute for professional medical advice, but they can make conversations with your oncologist or primary care provider more productive and focused. By equipping yourself with reliable information and structured tools, you become an active participant in your care, rather than a passive recipient of recommendations.

Above all, this book is an invitation to approach your journey with both curiosity and caution. The landscape of cancer treatment is evolving, and while new possibilities can inspire hope, they also demand discernment. By engaging with the material here, you are taking a thoughtful, measured step toward understanding options that may complement your established care. The hope is that, as you move through the chapters ahead, you will find not only knowledge but also reassurance—knowing that you are not alone in seeking answers, and that your efforts to advocate for yourself or your loved one are both valid and valued.

Your experience matters. Your questions are important. As you read on, may you find clarity, confidence, and a renewed sense of partnership in your care.

1.2 Disclaimer and Safe Use Notice

This book is intended as a comprehensive resource for patients and caregivers seeking to understand the reported use of fenbendazole and ivermectin in cancer care. It is essential to clarify from the outset that the information contained herein is for educational and informational purposes only. While every effort has been made to ensure accuracy, reliability, and clarity, this book does not constitute medical advice, diagnosis, or prescription. The protocols, insights, and patient experiences described are not a substitute for professional medical evaluation or treatment.

Cancer is a complex and multifaceted disease, and its management should always be guided by a qualified healthcare team. The reported uses of fenbendazole and ivermectin in oncology are still the subject of ongoing research and debate within the medical community. Although some patients and caregivers have chosen to explore these agents, such decisions must be approached with caution and under the direct supervision of a physician experienced in oncology. Self-administering medications—especially those not approved for human cancer treatment—can carry significant risks, including drug interactions, unexpected side effects, and interference with standard therapies.

Throughout this book, you will encounter summaries of published research, anecdotal reports, and practical tools designed to help you make sense of a rapidly evolving landscape. However, the inclusion of protocols or patient stories does not imply endorsement or guarantee of safety or efficacy. Regulatory agencies such as the U.S. Food and Drug Administration (FDA) and the European Medicines Agency (EMA) have not approved fenbendazole or ivermectin for the treatment of cancer in humans. Their use in this context remains *off-label* and experimental. Any decision to pursue these approaches should be made in close consultation with your oncologist or primary care provider, who can help assess potential benefits and risks in the context of your unique medical situation.

It is important to recognize that legal frameworks regarding the use of veterinary or non-standard medications in humans vary by country and region. Procuring, possessing, or using such substances outside of approved indications may have legal implications. This book does not provide guidance on sourcing, purchasing, or importing any medication. Readers are strongly advised to adhere to local laws and regulations, and to discuss any questions or intentions with their healthcare team before taking action.

The authors and publishers of this book have no financial interest in any product or protocol mentioned. Our sole aim is to provide a clear, balanced, and practical overview for those seeking to understand these emerging topics. We urge all readers to remain vigilant against misinformation, unverified claims, and sources that promise guaranteed results. Critical thinking and open communication with your medical team are your best safeguards.

In summary, this book is designed to empower you with knowledge, not to replace the expertise of your healthcare providers. Use the information here as a foundation for informed discussions, thoughtful questions, and collaborative decision-making. Your safety and well-being are paramount. Always prioritize professional guidance, and never hesitate to seek clarification or second opinions when considering any new approach to care.

1.3 How to Use This Handbook

Navigating a complex and often overwhelming landscape of information is a familiar challenge for those facing cancer, whether as patients or caregivers. This handbook is designed to serve as a clear, practical resource—one that can be approached in several ways, depending on your needs, background, and current stage of the journey. Understanding how to use this book effectively will help you extract the most relevant, actionable insights while avoiding confusion or misinterpretation.

Begin by considering your primary objectives. Some readers will seek a comprehensive understanding of the science behind fenbendazole and ivermectin, while others may be most interested in practical protocols, patient experiences, or tools for daily management. The structure of the book reflects these varied needs, with each part addressing a distinct aspect of the subject. If you are new to these compounds, the early chapters in Part II provide a solid foundation in the underlying research and evolving scientific context. These chapters distill complex studies into clear, accessible explanations, always with an eye toward clinical relevance and practical decision-making.

For those already familiar with the basics, the sections on reported protocols and patient practices offer a closer look at how individuals have incorporated these approaches into their care. Here, you will find not only descriptions of common regimens but also the rationale behind them, as well as real-world examples of how patients and caregivers have adapted protocols to their unique circumstances. This is not a prescriptive manual; rather, it is a compendium of reported strategies, presented with careful attention to both the potential benefits and the limitations or uncertainties that remain.

Safety and integration are central themes throughout the book. The chapters dedicated to these topics emphasize the importance of ongoing communication with your healthcare team and provide frameworks for discussing alternative or complementary approaches in a clinical setting. Checklists and planning tools are included to help you organize information, track progress, and prepare for meaningful conversations with your providers. These resources are designed to empower you as an informed participant in your care, supporting both autonomy and collaboration.

As you move through the book, you may wish to use the patient and caregiver stories as touchstones—sources of perspective and encouragement, as well as practical wisdom. These narratives illustrate the diversity of experiences and remind us that every journey is unique. They can also highlight questions or considerations you might not have anticipated, prompting deeper reflection or dialogue with your support network.

The reference tools and quick guides in the later chapters are intended for repeated consultation. Whether you are preparing for a new phase of treatment, reassessing your current approach, or simply seeking clarity on a specific point, these sections offer concise, actionable summaries. They are particularly useful for busy caregivers or patients managing multiple responsibilities, providing a way to access essential information quickly and efficiently.

Throughout the book, you will encounter a balance of scientific rigor and practical guidance. When interpreting research findings, pay close attention to the context in which studies were conducted, the strength of the evidence, and any noted limitations. Where uncertainty exists, it is clearly acknowledged, and readers are encouraged to approach new information with a critical, discerning mindset. This is especially important in a field where anecdotal reports and emerging data often intersect, sometimes leading to confusion or unrealistic expectations.

To make the most of this handbook, approach it as both a reference and a companion. Use it to clarify your understanding, to organize your questions, and to support ongoing dialogue with your healthcare team. Mark sections that are particularly relevant to your situation, and revisit them as your needs evolve. Remember that the information provided here is intended to supplement—not replace—professional medical advice. The most effective use of this resource is as a bridge: connecting you with the latest knowledge, practical tools, and the confidence to participate actively in your care decisions.

In summary, let this book serve as a structured, reliable guide through a rapidly changing landscape. By engaging with each section thoughtfully and critically, you equip yourself to navigate uncertainty with greater clarity, to advocate effectively for your needs, and to foster a collaborative, informed approach to care—whatever your path may hold.

CHAPTER 2: THE STORY BEHIND THE PROTOCOLS

2.1 THE ORIGINS OF INTEREST IN FENBENDAZOLE AND IVERMECTIN

The story of how fenbendazole and ivermectin, both originally developed as antiparasitic agents, became the focus of oncological interest is a compelling example of scientific curiosity intersecting with clinical need. These medications, long staples in veterinary and, in the case of ivermectin, also human medicine, were designed to address parasitic infections—fenbendazole for nematodes and cestodes in animals, and ivermectin for a range of human and animal parasites. Their mechanisms of action, targeting microtubule formation and chloride ion channels respectively, were well-characterized within their intended domains. Yet, the journey from barnyard to bedside, from deworming to potential anticancer applications, unfolded through a combination of serendipity, observation, and the persistent questioning that drives medical progress.

Interest in repurposing existing drugs for cancer is not new. The principle of drug repurposing—leveraging known safety profiles and pharmacology to accelerate the search for new treatments—has gained traction over the past two decades, particularly as the cost and time associated with developing novel oncology drugs have soared. Within this context, fenbendazole and ivermectin began to attract attention not from large pharmaceutical companies, but from researchers, clinicians, and, crucially, patients and caregivers searching for options beyond conventional protocols.

The earliest signals that fenbendazole might possess anticancer properties emerged from laboratory studies exploring its effects on cellular microtubules. Microtubules are essential for cell division, and their disruption is a well-established strategy in oncology, as seen with drugs like paclitaxel and vincristine. Researchers noted that fenbendazole, by binding to tubulin and destabilizing microtubules, could inhibit the proliferation of rapidly dividing cells—a hallmark of cancer. Initial in vitro studies, particularly those involving glioblastoma and other aggressive tumor cell lines, demonstrated reduced cell viability and increased apoptosis following fenbendazole exposure. These findings, while preliminary, provided a mechanistic rationale for further exploration.

Ivermectin's path to oncological interest followed a parallel yet distinct trajectory. Recognized globally for its transformative impact on parasitic diseases such as river blindness, ivermectin's broad biological activity led to investigations beyond antiparasitic effects. In the early 2010s, a series of preclinical studies began to reveal ivermectin's ability to modulate cellular signaling pathways implicated in cancer, including the inhibition of the WNT/β-catenin and PAK1 pathways, as well as the induction of cancer cell apoptosis. Notably, ivermectin appeared to exert selective toxicity against cancer cells while sparing normal cells, a property that fueled further investigation.

The historical context for this surge of interest cannot be overstated. As cancer patients and their families increasingly sought out integrative and complementary approaches, stories began to circulate—often via online forums and patient networks—about individuals experiencing unexpected improvements after self-administering fenbendazole or ivermectin. One widely publicized case involved a patient with advanced lung cancer who, after exhausting standard therapies, reported remarkable regression following fenbendazole use. While anecdotal and not a substitute for controlled clinical evidence, such stories captured the imagination of both the public and segments of the medical community, prompting calls for rigorous scientific evaluation.

This convergence of laboratory data, mechanistic plausibility, and patient-driven narratives created a unique momentum. Researchers began to publish case reports, small case series, and reviews summarizing the available evidence. At the same time, regulatory agencies and professional societies issued statements urging caution, emphasizing the need for robust clinical trials to establish efficacy and safety in cancer settings. The dialogue between patients, caregivers, and clinicians became more nuanced, with increasing recognition of the importance of clear communication, shared decision-making, and the responsible integration of emerging evidence.

Today, the interest in fenbendazole and ivermectin as potential adjuncts in cancer therapy reflects both the promise and the complexity of drug repurposing. The path from antiparasitic agent to experimental oncology protocol is neither linear nor complete; it is marked by ongoing research, evolving patient experiences, and the critical need for informed, collaborative decision-making. As the landscape continues to shift, understanding the origins of this interest provides essential context for evaluating current protocols, interpreting new data, and navigating the uncertainties inherent in integrative cancer care.

2.2 The Joe Tippens Case

In late 2016, Joe Tippens, a businessman from Oklahoma, received a diagnosis that would alter the course of his life and, eventually, spark a global conversation. He had been experiencing persistent symptoms—fatigue, unexplained weight loss, and a nagging cough—that led him to seek medical attention. The diagnosis was devastating: small cell lung cancer, already metastatic, with evidence of spread to his liver, pancreas, bladder, and bones. The prognosis was grim. According to his medical team, the expectation was a matter of months, not years, even with the best available therapies.

Tippens underwent standard-of-care treatments, including chemotherapy and radiation, which are the mainstays for aggressive cancers like his. Despite these interventions, his physicians made it clear that the disease's extent and biology left little room for optimism. Facing limited options, Tippens began searching for alternatives, determined to leave no stone unturned. It was during this period of research that he encountered an unusual thread on an online forum: anecdotal reports of cancer regression in laboratory animals treated with fenbendazole, a common veterinary anthelmintic used to treat parasitic infections in dogs.

The initial reports Tippens found were not from peer-reviewed journals but from informal discussions among researchers and pet owners. He learned of a scientist at Merck who, after being diagnosed with brain cancer, reportedly experienced remission after self-administering fenbendazole alongside conventional therapy. Intrigued by the possibility, Tippens reached out to this individual and, after gathering as much information as he could, decided to try the drug himself. He adopted a regimen that included fenbendazole, vitamin E, curcumin, and CBD oil, documenting his journey in detail.

Within several months, Tippens reported a remarkable turnaround. Follow-up imaging showed regression of his metastatic lesions, and eventually, his scans were interpreted as showing no evidence of active disease. Tippens attributed his recovery to the *fenbendazole protocol*, though he continued to acknowledge the role of prior chemotherapy and radiation. His story, shared on his blog and through social media, quickly gained traction. Patients and caregivers around the world began to take notice, and the phenomenon became a subject of intense discussion in online cancer communities.

The Tippens case is notable for several reasons. First, it highlights the profound impact that patient-driven narratives can have on the broader cancer landscape. While his experience is, by definition, anecdotal and cannot substitute for controlled clinical evidence, it catalyzed a wave of interest in repurposing veterinary drugs for human oncology. The story was picked up by mainstream media outlets and circulated widely, often with headlines that blurred the line between hope and hype. Tippens himself has consistently emphasized that he is not a physician and does not offer medical advice, but the sheer volume of correspondence he received from desperate patients underscores the hunger for new options among those facing advanced disease.

From a scientific perspective, the Tippens case underscores both the potential and the limitations of *real-world evidence*. While his remission is objectively documented, attributing causality to fenbendazole remains speculative. Small cell lung cancer is notoriously aggressive, and spontaneous remissions, while rare, are not impossible. Moreover, Tippens received standard therapies that may have contributed to his outcome. Nonetheless, his case prompted some clinicians and researchers to revisit the preclinical literature on fenbendazole and related compounds, exploring possible mechanisms such as microtubule disruption, interference with glucose metabolism, and modulation of cellular stress responses.

The media attention surrounding Tippens also brought to light important ethical and safety considerations. The use of non-approved drugs outside of clinical trials carries inherent risks, including unknown side effects, drug interactions, and the potential for patients to forgo established treatments. Regulatory agencies and professional societies responded by reiterating the importance of evidence-based medicine and the need for rigorous clinical studies before new protocols are adopted.

Yet, the Tippens story cannot be dismissed as mere anecdote. It reflects a broader movement within the patient community toward *empowerment* and active participation in treatment decisions. For many, his journey offers not just a template for exploring unconventional options, but also a reminder of the value of hope, curiosity, and critical inquiry. The ripple effects of his experience are evident in the increasing number of patients and caregivers who seek out information on fenbendazole and ivermectin, often arriving at their oncologist's office with detailed questions and a desire for open dialogue.

In sum, the Joe Tippens case stands as a pivotal moment in the evolving narrative of integrative oncology. It illustrates both the promise and the perils of patient-led innovation, the power of storytelling, and the ongoing need for collaboration between patients, clinicians, and researchers. As interest in repurposed drugs continues to grow, Tippens's journey serves as a compelling example of how individual experiences can shape the collective search for new answers in cancer care.

2.3 FROM ANECDOTE TO AWARENESS

As the first personal stories of unconventional cancer journeys began to surface, their impact was initially limited to small circles—family, friends, and perhaps a few local support groups. However, the digital age would soon transform these isolated anecdotes into a phenomenon of global awareness. The story of Joe Tippens, which had already begun to circulate among patients and caregivers seeking hope beyond conventional therapies, became a catalyst for a much broader movement. His account, detailed and persistent, was shared not only in person but across online forums, blogs, and eventually social media platforms with unprecedented reach.

The power of the internet to amplify individual voices cannot be overstated. Patient forums dedicated to specific cancers, such as lung or colorectal, became fertile ground for exchanging experiences and hypotheses. In these virtual spaces, stories about fenbendazole and later ivermectin were not merely recounted—they were dissected, debated, and, crucially, documented. The rise of Facebook groups, Reddit threads, and YouTube testimonials provided a platform where patients could connect across continents, compare notes, and build a collective narrative that extended far beyond any single individual. These communities, while diverse in background and geography, shared a common drive: to seek out new possibilities when standard options had been exhausted.

Media coverage soon followed, often drawn by the sheer volume and emotional resonance of these stories. Reports in mainstream outlets ranged from cautious curiosity to outright skepticism, but each mention fueled further discussion. The interplay between grassroots patient advocacy and media attention created a feedback loop—stories generated interest, which prompted more coverage, which in turn brought new voices into the conversation. This dynamic was particularly evident during periods of heightened public focus on drug repurposing, as occurred during the COVID-19 pandemic, when ivermectin entered the spotlight for reasons unrelated to oncology. The convergence of these narratives, though sometimes confusing, contributed to a heightened general awareness of off-label and repurposed drug use.

Within these online communities, a kind of informal peer review process developed. Patients and caregivers would share not only successes but also setbacks, side effects, and unanswered questions. This transparency, while not a substitute for rigorous clinical research, provided a level of detail and nuance often missing from anecdotal reports. Patterns began to emerge: certain dosing regimens, combinations with supplements, and methods for tracking symptoms and response. The collective wisdom of these groups often outpaced the available scientific literature, especially in areas where formal studies lagged behind patient innovation.

It is important to recognize that this transition from isolated anecdote to widespread awareness did not occur without challenges. The rapid spread of information—sometimes accurate, sometimes speculative—posed significant risks. Misinformation could circulate as easily as genuine insight, and the absence of regulatory oversight in online spaces meant that patients bore the burden of critical evaluation. Yet, for many, these communities offered something that traditional medical channels could not: validation, emotional support, and a sense of agency. The ability to ask questions, share experiences, and learn from others in real time provided a counterbalance to the isolation that often accompanies a cancer diagnosis.

Healthcare professionals, too, began to take notice. Some oncologists and researchers monitored these discussions to identify emerging trends or patient-reported outcomes that might warrant further investigation. Others expressed concern about the potential for harm, emphasizing the need for evidence-based practice. The dialogue between patients and professionals was, and remains, complex—marked by both tension and opportunity. In some cases, patient-driven awareness has prompted formal research initiatives or compassionate use protocols, illustrating the potential for grassroots advocacy to influence the broader landscape of cancer care.

Ultimately, the journey from anecdote to awareness is a testament to the interconnectedness of the modern world. Individual stories, once confined to the margins, now have the power to shape public discourse, inform research priorities, and influence the choices of patients and caregivers everywhere. This democratization of information comes with both promise and peril, demanding careful navigation and critical thinking. Yet it also underscores a fundamental truth: in the search for answers, the collective voice of patients can be as powerful as any single discovery.

PART II
UNDERSTANDING THE SCIENCE

CHAPTER 3: FENBENDAZOLE: WHAT THE RESEARCH SAYS

3.1 APPROVED USES AND SAFETY HISTORY

Fenbendazole occupies a distinctive place in the landscape of veterinary medicine, recognized for its well-established use as a broad-spectrum anthelmintic. Originally developed in the 1970s, fenbendazole's primary role has been the treatment and control of gastrointestinal parasites in a variety of animal species, including dogs, cats, horses, cattle, sheep, and even exotic animals. Regulatory agencies such as the U.S. Food and Drug Administration (FDA), the European Medicines Agency (EMA), and analogous authorities in other regions have approved fenbendazole for these specific uses, with detailed labeling that outlines its indications, dosing regimens, and species-specific considerations.

The safety profile of fenbendazole is one of the key reasons for its enduring presence in veterinary practice. Over more than four decades of widespread use, fenbendazole has demonstrated a high margin of safety when administered according to approved guidelines. In companion animals such as dogs and cats, it is commonly prescribed for routine deworming protocols, often as part of preventive health care. In livestock, fenbendazole is integral to herd management, helping to control parasitic burdens that can compromise animal health and agricultural productivity. Its use extends to zoo and wildlife medicine as well, where the need for reliable and safe anthelmintic agents is paramount.

Regulatory documentation and post-marketing surveillance have consistently supported the notion that fenbendazole, when used as directed, is associated with minimal adverse effects. The most commonly reported side effects are mild and transient, such as occasional gastrointestinal upset (vomiting or diarrhea) in sensitive animals. Serious adverse reactions are rare, and the drug's *therapeutic index*—the ratio between effective and potentially toxic doses—is considered wide. This characteristic has made fenbendazole a preferred choice among veterinarians, especially in situations where repeated or long-term administration is necessary.

The mechanism of action underlying fenbendazole's antiparasitic effect is well characterized. It belongs to the benzimidazole class of compounds, which exert their activity by binding to *β-tubulin* in parasitic worms, thereby disrupting microtubule formation and interfering with essential cellular functions. This targeted mechanism contributes to the selective toxicity of fenbendazole against parasites, while sparing the host animal's cells at therapeutic doses. The drug is typically administered orally, either as a tablet, paste, or suspension, and is known for its stability and ease of dosing across a range of animal sizes and species.

From a regulatory perspective, the approval process for fenbendazole involved rigorous evaluation of its efficacy, safety, and pharmacokinetics in target species. These data are publicly available in documents such as the FDA's New Animal Drug Application (NADA) summaries and EMA's European Public Assessment Reports (EPARs). These resources provide transparency regarding the studies conducted, the populations examined, and the observed outcomes, offering reassurance to veterinarians and animal owners alike.

It is important to emphasize that, to date, fenbendazole is not approved for use in humans by any major regulatory authority. Its use in human medicine remains investigational and is limited to specific research settings. The robust safety data accumulated from veterinary applications, however, have contributed to growing scientific interest in exploring its potential in other contexts, as discussed in later chapters.

In summary, fenbendazole's reputation as a safe and effective antiparasitic agent is built on decades of regulated use, extensive clinical experience, and a well-understood mechanism of action. Its track record in animal health provides a solid foundation for understanding both its benefits and its limitations. For those considering any off-label or investigational use, it is essential to recognize the boundaries of current regulatory approval and to approach new applications with a critical, evidence-based mindset.

3.2 Laboratory and Preclinical Studies

The scientific exploration of fenbendazole's potential in oncology has largely unfolded within the controlled environments of laboratories and animal models. These *preclinical studies* serve as the foundational step in evaluating any new therapeutic hypothesis, providing initial insights into mechanisms of action, efficacy, and safety before human trials are considered. In the case of fenbendazole, a drug originally developed for veterinary use against parasitic worms, its unexpected anticancer properties emerged from a combination of serendipitous observations and systematic inquiry.

Researchers first noted that fenbendazole's structure shares similarities with other benzimidazoles, a class known to disrupt microtubule formation in parasites. Microtubules are essential for cell division, and their disruption is a well-established target in cancer therapy—exemplified by drugs like vincristine and paclitaxel. This structural insight prompted scientists to test fenbendazole's effects on cancer cells in vitro, using cultured human and animal tumor cell lines. Across multiple studies, fenbendazole demonstrated the ability to inhibit cancer cell proliferation. For example, in lung cancer cell models, treatment with fenbendazole led to a marked reduction in cell viability, with evidence of cell cycle arrest and induction of apoptosis—a form of programmed cell death critical to preventing tumor growth.

The methodologies employed in these studies are rigorous and standardized. Typically, researchers expose cultured cancer cells to varying concentrations of fenbendazole, monitoring outcomes such as cell survival, changes in the cell cycle, and markers of apoptosis. Advanced techniques—such as flow cytometry, Western blotting for protein expression, and microscopy—are used to dissect the drug's impact at a molecular level. Notably, fenbendazole's effects are not limited to a single tumor type. Studies have reported activity against colorectal, breast, and prostate cancer cell lines, suggesting a broad mechanism of action potentially linked to the disruption of microtubule dynamics and interference with cellular metabolism.

Animal models provide the next layer of evidence, bridging the gap between cell culture and clinical application. In these experiments, human cancer cells are implanted into immunocompromised mice to create *xenograft* tumors. Fenbendazole is then administered, and researchers monitor tumor growth, animal survival, and potential side effects. Several studies have reported that mice receiving fenbendazole exhibit slower tumor progression compared to controls. In some cases, the drug appeared to enhance the effects of established chemotherapeutics, pointing to possible synergistic interactions. Importantly, these animal studies also monitor for toxicity, and fenbendazole has generally demonstrated a favorable safety profile at doses effective against tumors.

Despite these promising signals, it is essential to recognize the inherent limitations of laboratory and preclinical research. The controlled conditions of cell culture do not fully replicate the complexity of human tumors, which exist within a dynamic microenvironment influenced by the immune system, blood supply, and myriad signaling pathways. Similarly, while mouse models offer valuable insights, differences in metabolism and immune function mean that results do not always translate directly to humans. Furthermore, most preclinical studies utilize doses and administration schedules optimized for experimental outcomes, which may not reflect practical or safe regimens for patients.

Another important consideration is the publication bias that can affect the scientific literature. Positive findings are more likely to be reported than negative or inconclusive results, potentially skewing perceptions of efficacy. Additionally, many of the published studies on fenbendazole's anticancer effects are preliminary, with small sample sizes and limited replication. The lack of large-scale, independent validation means that these findings, while intriguing, must be interpreted with caution.

Nevertheless, the collective body of laboratory and preclinical evidence has established a credible scientific rationale for further investigation. Fenbendazole's ability to disrupt microtubule function, interfere with glucose metabolism, and induce apoptosis in a variety of cancer models positions it as a candidate for more advanced research. The next logical step would be carefully designed clinical trials to determine whether these laboratory observations can be translated into meaningful benefits for patients.

In summary, the laboratory and preclinical studies of fenbendazole have uncovered mechanisms that align with established principles of cancer biology and have demonstrated anticancer activity in controlled settings. These results provide a compelling, though preliminary, foundation for ongoing research. As with any promising therapy, the journey from bench to bedside is complex and requires rigorous validation, but the groundwork laid by these studies is an essential part of that process.

3.3 Reported Mechanisms of Action

Among the most discussed features of fenbendazole in the context of cancer research are its potential mechanisms of action at the cellular and molecular level. While the drug's established use in veterinary medicine targets parasitic microtubules, preclinical investigations have raised intriguing possibilities about its effects on human cancer cells—possibilities that remain, at present, largely theoretical and unproven in clinical settings.

The primary mechanism proposed for fenbendazole's anticancer activity centers on its interaction with *microtubules*, the dynamic protein structures essential for cell division. Microtubules form the mitotic spindle, which orchestrates the precise separation of chromosomes during mitosis. Fenbendazole belongs to the benzimidazole class, which is known to bind to β-tubulin subunits, thereby destabilizing microtubule assembly. In laboratory models, this disruption leads to mitotic arrest, followed by programmed cell death (apoptosis) in rapidly dividing cells—a hallmark of many cancer types. Notably, this mechanism is conceptually similar to that of established chemotherapeutics such as vincristine and paclitaxel, though fenbendazole's binding affinity and specificity differ. Studies such as those by Dogra et al. (2018) have demonstrated that fenbendazole can inhibit microtubule polymerization in cultured human cancer cell lines, resulting in cell cycle arrest at the G2/M phase.

Beyond its effects on microtubules, researchers have explored additional cellular pathways potentially influenced by fenbendazole. Some preclinical studies suggest that the drug may interfere with *glucose metabolism* in cancer cells. Tumor cells characteristically rely on high rates of glycolysis—a phenomenon known as the Warburg effect—to fuel their growth, even in the presence of oxygen. Fenbendazole has been reported to reduce the expression of glucose transporters (such as GLUT-4) and key glycolytic enzymes, thereby impairing glucose uptake and energy production in cancer cells. This metabolic disruption, observed in vitro, may sensitize tumor cells to oxidative stress and enhance their vulnerability to other treatments. However, these findings are preliminary and have not been validated in human subjects.

A further area of interest involves the drug's potential to modulate the *p53 tumor suppressor pathway*. The p53 protein plays a crucial role in maintaining genomic stability by inducing cell cycle arrest or apoptosis in response to DNA damage. Some laboratory studies have indicated that fenbendazole may upregulate p53 activity in certain cancer cell lines, thereby promoting apoptosis. This effect, while compelling in controlled environments, is not yet substantiated by in vivo or clinical data.

Additionally, fenbendazole's impact on *angiogenesis*—the formation of new blood vessels that supply nutrients to tumors—has been examined in animal models. There is limited evidence that the drug may inhibit angiogenic signaling pathways, potentially restricting tumor growth and metastasis. These anti-angiogenic effects, if confirmed, would align fenbendazole with a class of targeted therapies designed to starve tumors by cutting off their blood supply.

It is essential to underscore the distinction between these mechanistic hypotheses and established clinical evidence. The majority of data supporting these mechanisms derive from cell culture experiments and animal studies. While such preclinical research is invaluable for generating hypotheses and guiding further investigation, it does not equate to proven efficacy or safety in humans. The translation of laboratory findings to clinical benefit is a complex process, often marked by setbacks and unanticipated challenges.

Moreover, the doses and exposure times used in laboratory settings frequently differ from those achievable or safe in human patients. For example, concentrations of fenbendazole that disrupt microtubules in vitro may not be attainable in the human body without unacceptable toxicity. The pharmacokinetics and metabolism of fenbendazole in humans are not fully characterized, and its interactions with other medications—especially standard chemotherapeutic agents—remain largely unexplored.

In summary, the reported mechanisms of action for fenbendazole in cancer models include microtubule destabilization, disruption of glucose metabolism, modulation of the p53 pathway, and inhibition of angiogenesis. Each of these mechanisms is supported by varying degrees of preclinical evidence, but none have been confirmed in rigorous clinical trials involving cancer patients. As such, while the scientific rationale for further investigation exists, claims regarding fenbendazole's effectiveness in oncology must be tempered by the current lack of definitive human data. This distinction between laboratory promise and clinical reality is critical for patients and caregivers seeking to make informed, evidence-based decisions.

3.4 Shared Vulnerabilities Between Parasites and Tumor Cells

The scientific rationale for exploring antiparasitic agents like fenbendazole in oncology rests on a fascinating intersection of biology: the presence of **shared vulnerabilities between parasites and tumor cells**. At first glance, these two entities—one a multicellular invader, the other a rogue population of the body's own cells—might seem worlds apart. Yet, a closer look at their survival strategies reveals striking parallels that have drawn the attention of researchers seeking new therapeutic avenues.

Both parasites and cancer cells are, fundamentally, masters of adaptation. They thrive in hostile environments, evade immune detection, and hijack host resources to fuel their proliferation. This convergence is not coincidental. Evolution has equipped both with mechanisms to resist cell death, manipulate metabolic pathways, and, crucially, exploit the cytoskeletal machinery that underpins cell division and mobility.

Fenbendazole, a benzimidazole-class compound, was originally developed to target the *microtubules* of parasitic worms. Microtubules are dynamic protein structures essential for cell shape, intracellular transport, and, most notably, the segregation of chromosomes during mitosis. By binding to *β-tubulin*, fenbendazole disrupts the assembly of these structures, leading to the death of the parasite. Remarkably, cancer cells—especially those with high rates of division—are equally dependent on intact microtubule networks. This dependency creates an Achilles' heel: agents that destabilize microtubules in parasites can exert similar effects on tumor cells, halting their proliferation and triggering programmed cell death.

This shared vulnerability is not merely theoretical. The clinical success of established chemotherapeutics such as vincristine, vinblastine, and paclitaxel, all of which target microtubules, underscores the validity of this approach. What sets fenbendazole apart is its unique binding profile and low toxicity in mammalian cells at standard doses, as demonstrated in preclinical models. These properties have prompted a wave of laboratory studies investigating whether its antiparasitic action can translate into anticancer effects—an inquiry grounded in the biological commonalities between the two cell types.

Beyond microtubules, the metabolic flexibility of both parasites and cancer cells offers another point of intersection. Both must adapt to fluctuating nutrient supplies and oxidative stress within the host environment. Some parasites, for example, upregulate glycolysis—the breakdown of glucose for energy—in oxygen-poor conditions, a strategy mirrored by cancer cells in the well-known *Warburg effect*. This metabolic reprogramming is not just a survival tactic; it is a hallmark of aggressive tumor behavior. Certain antiparasitic drugs, including fenbendazole, have been shown in laboratory settings to interfere with glucose uptake and disrupt key metabolic enzymes. By targeting these conserved pathways, such agents may impair the ability of both parasites and tumor cells to thrive.

Another layer of similarity lies in how both parasites and cancer cells interact with the immune system. Parasites have evolved sophisticated mechanisms to dampen host immune responses, allowing them to persist undetected. Cancer cells, too, employ immune evasion tactics—downregulating surface markers, secreting immunosuppressive factors, and creating protective microenvironments. Some antiparasitic agents have demonstrated immunomodulatory effects, potentially reversing these evasive maneuvers and restoring the body's natural defenses against malignant cells.

The convergence of these biological characteristics explains why drugs like fenbendazole, designed for a completely different purpose, have entered the spotlight in oncology research. The concept is not without precedent: repurposing existing drugs based on shared cellular targets has yielded important breakthroughs in cancer therapy. However, it is essential to recognize that while laboratory findings are promising, translating these insights into clinical benefit requires rigorous validation.

In practical terms, understanding these shared vulnerabilities helps patients and caregivers appreciate the scientific logic behind the reported use of antiparasitic agents in cancer contexts. It also underscores the importance of critical evaluation and ongoing research. The parallels between parasites and tumor cells are compelling, but they are only one piece of a complex puzzle. As the field advances, the hope is that these insights will inform safer, more effective integrative strategies—always in concert with established medical care and under the guidance of informed healthcare professionals.

CHAPTER 4: IVERMECTIN: BEYOND ITS ORIGINAL PURPOSE

4.1 APPROVED USES IN HUMANS

Ivermectin's journey in human medicine began with a singular, transformative purpose: the treatment of parasitic diseases that, for decades, had caused immense suffering in some of the world's most vulnerable populations. Approved in the early 1980s, ivermectin quickly became a cornerstone of global health initiatives, particularly in regions where *onchocerciasis* (river blindness) and *lymphatic filariasis* were endemic. Its introduction marked a turning point in the fight against these debilitating conditions, offering a safe, effective, and easily administered therapy where few alternatives existed.

The primary approved indications for ivermectin in humans reflect its targeted antiparasitic action. In the United States and Europe, regulatory agencies such as the FDA and EMA have authorized ivermectin for the treatment of *strongyloidiasis*—an intestinal infection caused by the nematode *Strongyloides stercoralis*—and *onchocerciasis*, which is transmitted by blackflies and can lead to irreversible blindness. In these contexts, ivermectin's efficacy is well established, with decades of clinical use supporting its role as a first-line agent. The drug's mechanism—disrupting neural and muscular function in parasites by binding to glutamate-gated chloride channels—confers a high degree of selectivity, sparing human cells and minimizing systemic toxicity at approved doses.

Beyond these primary uses, ivermectin's label has expanded in some countries to include *scabies* and *head lice*, particularly when topical treatments fail or are impractical. Oral ivermectin, administered in carefully calculated doses, has demonstrated both safety and effectiveness in eradicating these infestations, providing relief for patients who might otherwise endure chronic discomfort and social stigma. The drug's oral formulation, ease of distribution, and favorable safety profile have made it a mainstay in mass drug administration campaigns, especially in resource-limited settings.

The global impact of ivermectin is difficult to overstate. The World Health Organization's endorsement of mass ivermectin distribution for river blindness and lymphatic filariasis has led to the treatment of hundreds of millions of individuals annually. These large-scale interventions have not only reduced the burden of disease but also contributed to the near-elimination of onchocerciasis in several countries. The safety record amassed through these programs is robust: adverse effects are generally mild and transient, most commonly including itching, mild swelling, or headache, often related to the body's response to dying parasites rather than the drug itself. Severe reactions are rare, and contraindications—such as use in children under 15 kg or in certain co-infections—are well defined and closely monitored.

In clinical practice, ivermectin is valued for its predictable pharmacokinetics, convenient single-dose regimens, and minimal drug-drug interactions at approved doses. Its oral administration bypasses many logistical barriers associated with injectable or topical therapies, further enhancing its utility in both individual patient care and public health campaigns. The drug's affordability and stability at room temperature have facilitated its inclusion on the World Health Organization's List of Essential Medicines, underscoring its central role in global health.

Despite its proven benefits, ivermectin's use remains circumscribed by regulatory frameworks that emphasize evidence-based indications. Off-label applications, while occasionally explored in clinical research or compassionate use scenarios, are not part of standard medical practice and require careful ethical and scientific consideration. The rigorous safety and efficacy standards governing ivermectin's approved uses serve as a model for the responsible integration of new therapies into medical care.

In summary, ivermectin's approved uses in human medicine are grounded in a substantial body of clinical evidence and real-world experience. Its role in combating parasitic diseases has been transformative, offering hope and tangible health gains to millions. The drug's safety, accessibility, and enduring effectiveness continue to make it a vital tool in the physician's armamentarium, while its story exemplifies the profound impact that targeted, evidence-based interventions can have on public health worldwide.

4.2 Cancer-Related Research

Interest in ivermectin as a potential anticancer agent has grown steadily over the past decade, propelled by a series of preclinical studies that have illuminated its multifaceted biological effects. Originally developed as an antiparasitic, ivermectin has demonstrated a surprising range of activities in laboratory models, including the ability to modulate key pathways involved in cancer cell survival and proliferation. This has led to a wave of research exploring its possible repositioning as an adjunct or alternative in oncology, particularly for patients facing limited options.

The bulk of the scientific literature to date centers on *preclinical investigations*—studies conducted in cell cultures and animal models. In these controlled environments, ivermectin has shown the capacity to inhibit cancer cell growth across a variety of tumor types, including lung, breast, colon, and glioblastoma. Mechanistically, researchers have observed that ivermectin can induce apoptosis (programmed cell death), inhibit cell cycle progression, and disrupt signaling pathways such as WNT/β-catenin and PAK1, both of which are implicated in tumor development and resistance to therapy. Notably, some studies have reported that ivermectin may also enhance the efficacy of certain chemotherapeutic agents, suggesting a possible *synergistic effect* when used in combination protocols.

Animal studies have provided further support for these findings. In murine models, ivermectin administration has been associated with reduced tumor growth and, in some cases, improved survival outcomes. For example, in mouse models of glioblastoma and breast cancer, treatment with ivermectin resulted in a measurable decrease in tumor volume, often without significant toxicity at the doses tested. These results have generated optimism about the drug's potential, particularly given its established safety profile in humans when used for approved indications.

However, the transition from laboratory findings to clinical application is a complex and often unpredictable process. At present, **clinical research involving ivermectin in oncology remains in its infancy**. Only a handful of early-phase trials have been registered or initiated, and published results are sparse. Most available data come from case reports or small, uncontrolled studies, which, while intriguing, do not provide the level of evidence required to support routine clinical use. For instance, isolated case reports have described patients with advanced cancers who experienced disease stabilization or partial responses while taking ivermectin, often in conjunction with other therapies. While these accounts are noteworthy, they are subject to significant limitations, including the absence of control groups, potential confounding factors, and the inherent variability of cancer progression.

The current research landscape is further complicated by the heterogeneity of study designs and patient populations. Dosing regimens, duration of treatment, and concomitant therapies vary widely across reports, making it difficult to draw definitive conclusions about efficacy or optimal use. Moreover, the underlying mechanisms by which ivermectin might exert anticancer effects in humans are not yet fully understood. While preclinical data provide compelling hypotheses, the translation of these effects to the clinical setting requires rigorous validation.

Importantly, the regulatory and ethical frameworks governing cancer research demand a high standard of evidence before new therapies can be recommended. As of now, **ivermectin is not approved for cancer treatment by any major health authority**, and its use in this context remains investigational. Patients and caregivers considering off-label use should be aware of these limitations and engage in open dialogue with their healthcare providers.

In summary, the scientific community has made significant strides in uncovering the potential anticancer properties of ivermectin, particularly through robust preclinical research. Yet, the **current clinical evidence is limited and inconclusive**, underscoring the need for well-designed clinical trials to clarify its role, if any, in oncology. Until such data are available, ivermectin's place in cancer care should be regarded as experimental, and decisions about its use should be made cautiously, with a clear understanding of the existing uncertainties and the guidance of experienced medical professionals.

4.3 Reported Mechanisms in Oncology Contexts

Within the scientific literature, ivermectin's potential in oncology has attracted growing interest, largely due to its multifaceted biological activity observed in preclinical studies. While originally developed as an antiparasitic agent, ivermectin has demonstrated a range of effects on cellular processes that are relevant to cancer biology. These reported mechanisms, though primarily described in laboratory models, provide a framework for understanding why some researchers and patients have considered ivermectin as an adjunct in cancer care.

One of the most frequently cited mechanisms involves the modulation of *cellular signaling pathways* that regulate cancer cell survival and proliferation. Ivermectin has been shown in vitro to inhibit the Wnt/β-catenin pathway—a critical driver of cell growth and differentiation in many tumor types. By interfering with this pathway, ivermectin may reduce the ability of cancer cells to multiply unchecked. In some experimental models, this effect translates to a decrease in tumor cell viability and, in certain cases, an increase in programmed cell death (apoptosis). It is important to emphasize that these findings are largely limited to cell cultures and animal models; translation to human disease remains under investigation.

Another area of interest is ivermectin's reported impact on *multidrug resistance* (MDR) in cancer cells. Many tumors develop resistance to chemotherapy by overexpressing efflux pumps—proteins that actively expel drugs from the cell, reducing their effectiveness. Ivermectin has been observed to inhibit some of these pumps, such as P-glycoprotein, in laboratory settings. This suggests a theoretical potential for ivermectin to enhance the efficacy of certain chemotherapeutic agents by allowing higher intracellular drug concentrations. However, clinical validation of this mechanism is still pending, and the complexity of MDR in human tumors poses significant challenges.

In addition to its effects on signaling and drug resistance, ivermectin has been reported to induce *cellular stress* within tumor cells. Some studies have documented the activation of pathways associated with oxidative stress and endoplasmic reticulum (ER) stress, both of which can compromise cancer cell survival. For example, increased reactive oxygen species (ROS) generation has been observed following ivermectin exposure, potentially tipping the balance toward cell death in already vulnerable tumor cells. These findings, while promising, must be interpreted with caution, as the same mechanisms could also affect healthy cells, underscoring the importance of careful dosing and monitoring.

A further proposed mechanism relates to ivermectin's interaction with the immune system. Preclinical research has indicated that ivermectin may modulate the tumor microenvironment, potentially enhancing the activity of immune cells such as cytotoxic T lymphocytes. Some animal studies suggest that ivermectin can reduce immunosuppressive signals within tumors, thereby supporting the body's natural anti-tumor defenses. This immunomodulatory effect is of particular interest in the era of immunotherapy, where the interplay between cancer and the immune system is a central focus of drug development.

It is also worth noting that ivermectin's ability to disrupt *ion channels*—specifically, chloride channels—has been implicated in its anticancer activity. By altering the flow of ions across cellular membranes, ivermectin may disturb the electrical balance required for cancer cell function and survival. While this mechanism is well-established in the context of its antiparasitic action, its relevance in oncology is still being elucidated.

Despite these intriguing findings, the transition from laboratory research to clinical application is fraught with complexity. The concentrations of ivermectin required to achieve these effects in cell cultures are often higher than those safely attainable in humans. Furthermore, the tumor microenvironment in patients is vastly more complex than what can be replicated in vitro or in animal models. As such, while the reported mechanisms offer a scientific rationale for ongoing research, they do not constitute proof of efficacy in humans.

In summary, ivermectin's reported anticancer mechanisms span several domains: inhibition of key signaling pathways, reversal of multidrug resistance, induction of cellular stress, modulation of immune responses, and disruption of ion channel function. Each of these mechanisms is supported by varying degrees of preclinical evidence, and together they form the basis for the current interest in ivermectin as a potential adjunct in oncology. However, it is essential to approach these findings with measured optimism, recognizing the gap that remains between laboratory promise and clinical reality. For patients and caregivers considering integrative approaches, these mechanistic insights can inform meaningful discussions with healthcare providers, fostering a shared understanding of both the possibilities and the limitations inherent in current research.

CHAPTER 5: THE CURRENT RESEARCH LANDSCAPE

5.1 WHAT WE KNOW VS. WHAT WE DON'T

The scientific landscape surrounding fenbendazole and ivermectin in oncology is characterized by a dynamic interplay between established facts, emerging hypotheses, and significant gaps in knowledge. To navigate this complex terrain, it is essential to distinguish what is currently supported by credible research from what remains speculative or uncertain.

Fenbendazole, a benzimidazole-class anthelmintic, has garnered attention due to laboratory studies suggesting anti-cancer properties. In vitro experiments—those conducted on cancer cell lines in controlled environments—have demonstrated that fenbendazole can disrupt microtubule formation, interfere with glucose metabolism, and induce apoptosis in certain cancer cells. These mechanistic insights provide a plausible biological rationale for further investigation. However, it is crucial to recognize that these findings are largely preclinical. To date, there are no published, peer-reviewed clinical trials in humans that establish fenbendazole's safety or efficacy as an anti-cancer agent. The evidence remains limited to laboratory and animal studies, which, while informative, cannot be directly extrapolated to patient care without rigorous human data.

Ivermectin, originally developed as an anti-parasitic agent, has also entered the oncology conversation. Its established safety profile in humans for approved indications has made it a candidate for repurposing. Preclinical research has identified several mechanisms by which ivermectin may exert anti-tumor effects, including modulation of cell signaling pathways, inhibition of cancer stem cells, and enhancement of immune responses. Some observational and case reports have described anecdotal benefits in cancer patients, but these are not substitutes for controlled clinical studies. As with fenbendazole, robust evidence from randomized controlled trials is lacking. The current body of knowledge is insufficient to support routine use of ivermectin in oncology outside of clinical trials.

What is known, therefore, is primarily rooted in laboratory science and early-stage research. Both agents have demonstrated intriguing biological activity against cancer cells in vitro and, to a lesser extent, in animal models. Their established pharmacological profiles in other contexts provide a foundation for considering repurposing. However, the translation from bench to bedside is fraught with challenges. The absence of well-designed clinical trials means that questions about optimal dosing, potential interactions with standard therapies, long-term safety, and true efficacy in human cancer remain unanswered.

Areas of uncertainty are substantial. The variability in reported patient experiences—ranging from perceived benefits to lack of effect or adverse events—reflects both the heterogeneity of cancer itself and the lack of standardized protocols. The potential for drug interactions, especially in patients undergoing complex oncologic regimens, is not well-characterized. Furthermore, the risk of self-medication or unsupervised use cannot be overstated, as it may lead to unforeseen complications or delays in evidence-based care.

The research landscape is evolving, with ongoing studies aiming to clarify the role of these agents in oncology. Some early-phase clinical trials are underway, but results are pending and should be interpreted with caution when they become available. Until more definitive data emerge, the use of fenbendazole and ivermectin in cancer should be regarded as experimental, and any consideration of these approaches must be grounded in transparent communication with healthcare professionals.

In summary, the current state of knowledge is defined by promising laboratory findings and a compelling rationale for further study, balanced by a clear recognition of the limitations and unknowns. The distinction between what is known and what remains to be discovered is not merely academic; it is central to informed, responsible decision-making for patients and caregivers navigating complex choices in oncology.

5.2 Ongoing and Planned Clinical Trials

The current research landscape for fenbendazole and ivermectin in oncology is characterized by a cautious but growing interest, particularly as anecdotal reports and preclinical findings have prompted formal investigation. Clinical trials represent the gold standard for evaluating both efficacy and safety, and the transition from laboratory studies to human trials is a significant milestone. However, it is essential to approach the subject with precision: as of this writing, the number of registered, actively recruiting clinical trials specifically assessing fenbendazole or ivermectin in cancer patients remains limited, reflecting both regulatory caution and the complexities of drug repurposing.

For fenbendazole, the clinical trial landscape is still in its infancy. Despite substantial online interest and a proliferation of patient-reported experiences, only a handful of studies have moved beyond the preclinical stage. The most notable is a Phase I trial registered in the United States, designed to evaluate the safety, tolerability, and pharmacokinetics of fenbendazole in patients with advanced solid tumors. This trial, listed on ClinicalTrials.gov (NCT number available via the registry), aims to establish foundational data regarding dosing and adverse effects, without yet addressing efficacy as a primary endpoint. Recruitment for this study is ongoing, and updates—including protocol amendments and interim safety findings—are typically published directly on the ClinicalTrials.gov entry. It is worth noting that other planned studies, particularly in Europe and Asia, are in earlier stages of protocol development or awaiting regulatory approval, and their details may be found in regional registries such as the EU Clinical Trials Register (EudraCT) or the Chinese Clinical Trial Registry.

Ivermectin, by contrast, has advanced somewhat further along the clinical research pathway, owing in part to its established safety profile in humans for antiparasitic indications. Several Phase II trials are underway or recently completed, exploring ivermectin as an adjunct to standard chemotherapy or immunotherapy in various malignancies, including glioblastoma, breast cancer, and colorectal cancer. These studies generally focus on endpoints such as progression-free survival, tumor response rates, and quality of life metrics. For example, a multicenter trial in South America is evaluating ivermectin in combination with temozolomide for recurrent glioblastoma, while another in Europe investigates its use alongside conventional regimens in metastatic breast cancer. Each trial is registered with a unique identifier, and readers can access up-to-date information—including eligibility criteria, enrollment status, and published results—through platforms like ClinicalTrials.gov, EudraCT, and the World Health Organization International Clinical Trials Registry Platform (ICTRP).

It is important to recognize that the majority of these trials remain in early phases, primarily designed to assess safety, optimal dosing, and preliminary signals of efficacy. The transition to larger, randomized Phase III studies will depend on the outcomes of these initial investigations. Until such data are available, any off-label use of fenbendazole or ivermectin for cancer should be approached with caution and always under the supervision of a qualified healthcare professional.

For patients and caregivers seeking to monitor the progress of these trials, institutional registries are the most reliable sources of information. ClinicalTrials.gov, maintained by the U.S. National Library of Medicine, offers comprehensive listings of ongoing and completed studies worldwide. The EudraCT database provides details for trials conducted within the European Union, while the ICTRP aggregates data from multiple national registries. These platforms are updated regularly and include essential information such as trial objectives, phase, recruitment status, contact information for study coordinators, and links to published results or press releases.

In summary, while the clinical trial landscape for fenbendazole and ivermectin in oncology is still emerging, it is marked by a methodical, evidence-driven approach. The number of ongoing and planned studies is steadily increasing, reflecting both scientific curiosity and patient demand. However, the field remains in a phase of cautious exploration, and the most authoritative updates will always be found in official trial registries and peer-reviewed publications. For those navigating this evolving terrain, staying informed through institutional sources is essential for making evidence-based decisions in collaboration with the healthcare team.

5.3 How to Interpret Scientific Studies

Interpreting scientific studies is an essential skill for anyone navigating complex medical decisions, particularly when considering integrative or off-label therapies. The landscape of cancer research is vast and often daunting, filled with studies of varying quality, intent, and reliability. Understanding how to critically evaluate this evidence empowers patients and caregivers to make informed choices, ask meaningful questions, and avoid common pitfalls. The following step-by-step guide demystifies the process, offering a clear path through the technical language and methodological nuances that define modern clinical research.

How to Critically Evaluate Scientific Studies

Overview: This process enables you to assess the credibility, relevance, and limitations of research studies, helping you distinguish robust evidence from weak or misleading claims.

Time Required: 15–30 minutes per study | **Difficulty:** Moderate

What You'll Need:

- Access to the full text of the study (not just the abstract)
- A notepad or digital document for notes
- Basic understanding of medical terminology (a glossary may be helpful)
- A critical mindset and willingness to question assumptions

Instructions:

Step 1: Identify the Level of Evidence

- Begin by determining what type of study you are reading. Is it a randomized controlled trial (RCT), a cohort study, a case series, a laboratory (in vitro) experiment, or a review article?
- The *hierarchy of evidence* places systematic reviews and meta-analyses at the top, followed by RCTs, observational studies, case reports, and, at the base, preclinical (animal or cell) studies.

• Recognizing the study type helps you understand how much weight to give its conclusions. For example, a single case report of fenbendazole use in cancer is far less conclusive than a large, well-designed clinical trial.

Step 2: Examine the Study's Endpoints

• Every study sets out to answer specific questions, known as *endpoints*. These may be *primary* (the main outcome, such as overall survival) or *secondary* (additional outcomes, like quality of life or tumor shrinkage).

• Scrutinize whether the endpoints are clinically meaningful. For instance, a reduction in tumor size (a surrogate endpoint) does not always translate into longer survival or improved well-being.

• Consider whether the endpoints were pre-specified or chosen after the data was collected—post hoc endpoints can introduce bias.

Step 3: Assess Study Design and Sample Size

• Evaluate how the study was structured. Was it randomized and blinded? Did it include a control group? These features reduce the risk of bias and increase reliability.

• Examine the *sample size*. Small studies are more prone to random error and may not represent the broader patient population.

• Look for details on how participants were selected and whether the groups were comparable at baseline. Imbalances can skew results.

Step 4: Look for Sources of Bias

• Bias can creep into studies at many stages: selection of participants, measurement of outcomes, data analysis, and reporting.

• Common types include *selection bias* (non-random assignment), *performance bias* (differences in care apart from the intervention), and *publication bias* (only positive results are published).

• Transparent studies will discuss their limitations and efforts to minimize bias. Be wary of studies that do not acknowledge these issues.

STEP 5: EVALUATE STATISTICAL SIGNIFICANCE AND CLINICAL RELEVANCE

• Statistical significance (often reported as a *p-value* less than 0.05) suggests that observed differences are unlikely due to chance. However, statistical significance does not always mean the result is important in practice.

• Consider the *effect size*—how large and meaningful is the difference? A therapy that improves survival by a few days may not justify risks or costs.

• Confidence intervals provide additional context, indicating the range within which the true effect likely falls.

STEP 6: SCRUTINIZE THE STUDY'S LIMITATIONS

• No study is perfect. Robust research will openly discuss its own limitations, such as small sample size, short follow-up, or lack of generalizability.

• Pay attention to conflicts of interest and funding sources. Studies sponsored by parties with a financial stake may be more likely to report favorable outcomes.

• Note whether the study's findings have been replicated independently. Single studies, especially those with surprising results, should be interpreted cautiously until confirmed by others.

TROUBLESHOOTING:

• **Issue:** The study only reports positive outcomes, with no mention of adverse effects or limitations. → **Solution:** Treat such studies with skepticism; balanced research discusses both benefits and risks.

• **Issue:** The study uses complex statistics without clear explanation. → **Solution:** Seek out plain-language summaries or consult a knowledgeable healthcare professional for interpretation.

• **Issue:** The study's sample is very small or highly selective. → **Solution:** Recognize that results may not apply broadly and look for larger, more diverse studies.

RED FLAGS AND COMMON PITFALLS

Certain warning signs should prompt extra caution. These include studies published in journals with questionable reputations, lack of peer review, or results that seem "too good to be true." Beware of studies that make sweeping claims based on laboratory findings alone, as results in cell cultures or animal models rarely translate directly to human benefit. Pay attention to overreliance on surrogate endpoints, selective reporting of outcomes, and absence of transparent methodology.

NEXT STEPS:

After critically appraising a study, integrate its findings with the broader body of evidence. Compare results across multiple studies and consider how they align—or conflict—with established knowledge. Use your notes to prepare thoughtful questions for your healthcare team, ensuring that any decisions about integrative or complementary therapies are grounded in the most reliable information available.

Mastering the art of interpreting scientific studies is not just an academic exercise; it is a vital tool for navigating uncertainty and becoming an active participant in your care. By applying these steps consistently, you will be better equipped to discern credible evidence, avoid common traps, and make decisions that reflect both the science and your individual values.

PART III
REPORTED PROTOCOLS AND PATIENT PRACTICES

CHAPTER 6: REPORTED USES AND APPROACHES

6.1 COMMONLY SHARED FENBENDAZOLE PROTOCOL PATTERNS

For patients and caregivers exploring reported fenbendazole protocols, clarity and structure are essential. The landscape is marked by anecdotal experiences, online communities, and a growing but still limited body of published research. This step-by-step guide synthesizes commonly shared patterns, aiming to provide a transparent overview of how individuals have approached fenbendazole use in oncological contexts. It is crucial to recognize that these protocols are not medically validated treatments for cancer, and all decisions should be made in close consultation with a qualified healthcare provider. The following process is intended to inform, not to recommend or endorse, any specific regimen.

FENBENDAZOLE PROTOCOL: COMMONLY REPORTED PATTERNS

Overview: This guide outlines the typical steps and considerations reported by patients who have chosen to incorporate fenbendazole into their regimen, including dosing patterns, monitoring strategies, and key safety precautions.

Time Required: Ongoing, with initial setup in 1–2 days | **Difficulty:** Moderate (requires careful tracking and communication with healthcare providers)

WHAT YOU'LL NEED:

- Pharmaceutical-grade fenbendazole (commonly 222 mg powder sachets or tablets, as found in veterinary formulations)
- Accurate digital scale (if dosing adjustments are needed)
- Personal health journal or tracking app
- Baseline laboratory results (liver function, blood counts)
- Support from a healthcare provider familiar with your case

INSTRUCTIONS:

STEP 1: ESTABLISH BASELINE HEALTH AND MEDICAL OVERSIGHT

• Schedule a consultation with your oncologist or primary physician to discuss your interest in fenbendazole. Present your rationale, and request baseline blood work, especially liver function tests and complete blood counts.

• This step is critical to ensure you are medically stable and to establish a point of comparison for ongoing monitoring.

• Success is a clear, documented baseline and explicit physician awareness of your intentions.

STEP 2: SELECT A DOSING PATTERN

• The most commonly reported regimen is 222 mg of fenbendazole daily for three consecutive days, followed by four days off (the so-called "3-on, 4-off" cycle). Some individuals report continuous daily dosing, while others use alternate-day schedules.

• Select a pattern based on your health status, previous experiences, and after discussing with your physician. Always start with the lowest effective dose, especially if you have pre-existing liver or kidney concerns.

• Ensure you are using a product free from potentially harmful excipients, and verify the source for quality assurance.

STEP 3: BEGIN ADMINISTRATION AND MONITOR CLOSELY

• Take fenbendazole orally, typically with food to enhance absorption and reduce the risk of gastrointestinal discomfort.

• Record each dose, time of administration, and any side effects or changes in symptoms in your health journal.

• Monitor for common side effects, which may include mild gastrointestinal upset, changes in stool, or, rarely, allergic reactions. Severe symptoms (jaundice, persistent nausea, unexplained fatigue) require immediate medical attention.

• Weekly or biweekly blood tests are advisable during the first month, focusing on liver enzymes and blood counts.

STEP 4: ADJUST AND INTEGRATE WITH OTHER THERAPIES

- Many patients report using fenbendazole alongside conventional therapies or supplements (see Chapter 7 for details on supportive measures). Document all concurrent medications and supplements to avoid potential interactions.
- If you experience side effects or laboratory abnormalities, pause the protocol and consult your physician before resuming or adjusting the dose.
- Success is defined by tolerability, absence of significant adverse effects, and ongoing medical supervision.

TROUBLESHOOTING:

- **Issue:** Gastrointestinal discomfort → **Solution:** Take with food, reduce dose, or extend off-days.
- **Issue:** Elevated liver enzymes → **Solution:** Discontinue immediately and seek medical evaluation.
- **Issue:** Uncertainty about product quality → **Solution:** Use only pharmaceutical-grade sources, avoid unverified online vendors.

Next Steps: After 4–6 weeks, review your progress with your healthcare provider. Reassess laboratory values, symptom changes, and overall tolerability. Adjust the protocol if necessary, or discontinue if adverse effects outweigh perceived benefits.

It is important to recognize that reported protocols are not standardized or universally accepted within the medical community. Variations exist in dosing frequency, duration, and combination with other agents. Some individuals, for example, incorporate intermittent "drug holidays" to minimize toxicity, while others adjust based on personal response or evolving laboratory results. Regardless of the pattern chosen, the foundation of any approach should be *open communication with your healthcare team, diligent self-monitoring, and a willingness to adapt based on emerging evidence and personal health status.*

Ultimately, the decision to explore fenbendazole protocols is deeply personal and often arises from a desire for agency in the face of limited options. By following a structured, safety-first approach, patients and caregivers can reduce uncertainty and maintain a proactive, informed stance within their broader care journey.

6.2 Commonly Shared Ivermectin Use Patterns

Interest in ivermectin as a potential adjunct in cancer care has grown in recent years, largely fueled by anecdotal reports and emerging preclinical research. For patients and caregivers navigating this landscape, understanding the commonly shared patterns of ivermectin use is essential—not only for clarity, but also for safety and effective communication with healthcare providers. While rigorous clinical data in oncology are still limited, publicly available sources and patient communities have reported a range of approaches. The following step-by-step guide synthesizes these patterns, highlighting practical considerations, common variants, and critical safety measures.

Ivermectin Use Patterns in Cancer Support

Overview: This process outlines the reported methods for using ivermectin in integrative cancer protocols, including dosing schedules, monitoring strategies, and essential precautions.

Time Required: Varies (typically 1–3 months per cycle, with ongoing assessment) | **Difficulty:** Moderate (requires careful attention to detail and medical oversight)

What You'll Need:

- Pharmaceutical-grade ivermectin (oral tablet or liquid, as prescribed or sourced)
- Accurate dosing tool (milligram scale or calibrated syringe for liquids)
- Patient logbook or digital tracker for dose, timing, and side effects
- Access to recent laboratory results (liver and kidney function, complete blood count)
- Direct line of communication with a healthcare professional

Instructions:

Step 1: Establish Baseline and Medical Oversight

- Consult your oncologist or primary care physician before initiating any off-label use of ivermectin. Share your intentions, obtain baseline bloodwork (liver enzymes, renal function, CBC), and discuss potential drug interactions.

• This step is crucial for identifying contraindications and establishing a point of reference for monitoring safety.

• Success is defined by clear, documented communication with your care team and a green light to proceed.

STEP 2: DETERMINE STARTING DOSE AND SCHEDULE

• Review publicly available protocols. The most commonly cited starting dose in patient forums and some published case reports is 0.2 mg/kg, administered orally once daily or every other day. For a 70 kg adult, this equates to approximately 14 mg per dose.

• Some individuals adjust frequency—using a "5 days on, 2 days off" pattern, or alternating weeks—based on tolerance and response.

• Begin with the lowest effective dose, especially if combining with other medications or supplements. Escalation should only occur under medical supervision.

• Be aware that over-the-counter veterinary formulations may differ in concentration and purity; pharmaceutical-grade human formulations are strongly preferred.

STEP 3: MONITOR FOR SIDE EFFECTS AND EFFICACY

• Document each dose, time of administration, and any symptoms in your logbook. Common side effects include mild gastrointestinal upset, dizziness, or skin rash. Rare but serious events (such as vision changes, confusion, or severe allergic reaction) require immediate medical attention.

• Monitor laboratory values at least every 2–4 weeks, or as advised by your physician. Look for changes in liver or kidney function, blood counts, or unexpected symptoms.

• Success is ongoing tolerance without significant adverse effects and stable laboratory parameters.

STEP 4: ADJUST PROTOCOL AS NEEDED

• If mild side effects occur, consider dose reduction or increasing the interval between doses. Some patients report improved tolerance with evening dosing or taking ivermectin with food.

- If laboratory abnormalities or moderate-to-severe side effects develop, discontinue use and consult your physician promptly. Never attempt to self-manage severe reactions.
- Regularly reassess the protocol with your care team, especially if starting new medications or supplements.

TROUBLESHOOTING:

- **Issue:** Nausea or stomach upset → **Solution:** Take with a small meal or reduce dose; monitor symptoms closely.
- **Issue:** Fatigue or dizziness → **Solution:** Lower dose or increase dosing interval; ensure adequate hydration.
- **Issue:** Laboratory abnormalities (elevated liver enzymes, low white blood cell count) → **Solution:** Discontinue ivermectin and seek medical evaluation immediately.

Next Steps: After completing a cycle (typically 4–8 weeks), review progress with your physician. Evaluate symptom changes, laboratory results, and overall well-being. Decide jointly whether to continue, pause, or discontinue the protocol. Always document your experiences to inform future decisions and discussions.

It is important to note that while these patterns are widely shared in patient communities, they are not substitutes for individualized medical advice. Variants exist: some protocols combine ivermectin with other agents (such as fenbendazole or supplements), while others adjust dosing based on side effect profiles or concurrent therapies. Integration with conventional care and consistent medical oversight remain the cornerstones of safety.

For many, this process represents a proactive step in exploring integrative options. It is natural to feel both hope and uncertainty. By following structured, transparent protocols and maintaining open communication with healthcare professionals, patients and caregivers can navigate this complex terrain with greater confidence and clarity.

6.3 Combination Strategies Patients Have Tried

In the landscape of reported off-label use, combination strategies involving fenbendazole and ivermectin have emerged as a frequent topic of discussion among patients and caregivers seeking integrative approaches. While robust clinical data are lacking, patient communities have shared a variety of practical methods for sequencing, timing, and monitoring these agents alongside other supportive measures. The following step-by-step guide synthesizes these reported practices, highlighting essential considerations for safety, documentation, and communication with healthcare professionals.

Combination Protocol Planning

Overview: This process helps structure the use of fenbendazole and ivermectin in combination, aiming to maximize potential synergy while minimizing risks and ensuring clear documentation.

Time Required: 30–60 minutes for initial planning, with ongoing daily monitoring | **Difficulty:** Moderate

What You'll Need:

- Written list of all current medications and supplements
- Access to a medication interaction checker (online or via pharmacist)
- A dedicated journal or digital log for tracking
- Support from a caregiver or family member, if possible
- Contact information for your healthcare team

Instructions:

Step 1: Map Out All Current Therapies

- Begin by listing every medication, supplement, and integrative therapy currently in use, including dosing and timing.
- This baseline inventory is essential for identifying potential interactions and overlaps. It also provides a foundation for communicating with your care team.

STEP 2: REVIEW REPORTED COMBINATION SEQUENCES

• Patients commonly report two main sequencing strategies: *alternating* (e.g., fenbendazole on certain days, ivermectin on others) and *concurrent* (both agents taken together, often at different times of day).

• Consider your own tolerance, previous experiences, and any guidance from your healthcare provider. For example, some individuals report taking fenbendazole in the morning and ivermectin in the evening to reduce gastrointestinal discomfort.

• Document your planned sequence clearly, noting start dates, days of administration, and any planned breaks.

STEP 3: ASSESS TIMING AND DOSING WINDOWS

• Determine optimal timing based on reported experiences and your daily routine. Many patients choose to align dosing with meals to minimize stomach upset, though some protocols recommend taking certain agents away from food for better absorption.

• If integrating with conventional therapies (such as chemotherapy), consult your oncologist about potential scheduling conflicts or synergies. Some patients opt to pause these agents during intensive treatment weeks to avoid compounding side effects.

• Clearly record your intended timing and rationale in your log.

STEP 4: CHECK FOR INTERACTIONS AND OVERLAPS

• Using your medication list, run a thorough interaction check—either with a reputable online tool or, preferably, with a pharmacist.

• Pay special attention to medications metabolized by the liver (notably CYP450 enzymes), as both fenbendazole and ivermectin may influence these pathways.

• If taking supplements such as antioxidants, probiotics, or immune modulators, cross-reference for possible antagonistic effects or absorption issues.

• Note any potential concerns and flag them for discussion with your healthcare provider.

STEP 5: DEFINE CRITERIA FOR PAUSING OR STOPPING

• Establish clear, personalized criteria for when to pause or discontinue one or both agents. Common triggers include new or worsening side effects (e.g., persistent nausea, rash, neurological symptoms), abnormal laboratory results, or advice from your medical team.

• Some patients use a "three-strike" rule—pausing after three consecutive days of moderate side effects, or immediately for any severe reaction.

• Document these criteria in your protocol log and share them with a caregiver for additional oversight.

STEP 6: TRACK AND DOCUMENT DAILY

• Each day, record doses taken, timing, any side effects, and subjective observations (energy, appetite, mood).

• Use a simple scale (e.g., 0–10) for symptoms and side effects to facilitate pattern recognition over time.

• Update your log with any changes to the protocol, missed doses, or new medications.

STEP 7: PREPARE DOCUMENTATION FOR YOUR HEALTHCARE TEAM

• Summarize your protocol, including agents, doses, timing, and rationale, in a concise format for your next medical appointment.

• Bring your daily log or a summary of key trends (side effects, improvements, concerns).

• Be prepared to discuss your decision-making process, criteria for pausing, and any questions about interactions or monitoring.

TROUBLESHOOTING:

• **Issue:** Unexpected side effects (e.g., dizziness, allergic reaction) → **Solution:** Pause both agents immediately, document the event, and contact your healthcare provider.

• **Issue:** Difficulty tracking doses or symptoms → **Solution:** Use a pill organizer, set phone reminders, or enlist caregiver support for daily logging.

- **Issue:** Uncertainty about interactions with new medications → **Solution:** Always check with your pharmacist or healthcare provider before adding new agents.

Next Steps: After two to four weeks, review your log for trends and meet with your healthcare team to assess safety, tolerability, and any observed effects. Adjust your protocol as needed, always prioritizing open communication and shared decision-making.

Combination strategies, when approached methodically, can offer a sense of agency and structure for patients navigating uncertain terrain. While these protocols are not substitutes for evidence-based oncology care, careful planning, ongoing documentation, and proactive communication with medical professionals can help mitigate risks and support more informed, collaborative decisions. As research evolves, maintaining a detailed record of your experiences may also contribute valuable data to the broader understanding of these emerging integrative approaches.

6.4 Why Experiences Differ

Outcomes reported by patients and caregivers using fenbendazole and ivermectin protocols are strikingly variable. This diversity is not random; it reflects the complex interplay of biological, practical, and contextual factors that shape each individual's experience. Understanding why responses differ is essential for setting realistic expectations, interpreting anecdotal reports, and making informed decisions about integrating these approaches into a broader care plan.

The first and most significant factor is the *biological individuality* of each patient and their cancer. Tumors are not uniform entities; they vary widely in origin, genetic mutations, growth rate, and how they interact with the body's immune system. For example, a patient with a slow-growing, well-differentiated tumor may experience a different response than someone facing an aggressive, metastatic cancer. Even within the same cancer type, genetic mutations such as KRAS, EGFR, or TP53 can influence how tumor cells respond to agents like fenbendazole or ivermectin. The underlying health of the patient, including liver and kidney function, immune status, and other comorbidities, further modulates how these substances are metabolized and tolerated.

The *stage of disease* at the time of protocol initiation is another critical variable. Early-stage cancers, with lower tumor burden and less systemic involvement, may be more responsive to interventions that target cellular metabolism or microtubule dynamics, mechanisms proposed for both fenbendazole and ivermectin. In contrast, advanced-stage cancers often exhibit greater heterogeneity, resistance mechanisms, and impaired organ function, all of which can blunt the effects of any adjunctive therapy. Timing matters: some patients start these protocols while still responding to standard treatments, others after exhausting all conventional options. The context in which these agents are introduced can profoundly influence both perceived and measurable outcomes.

Adherence to protocol is a practical yet powerful determinant of results. Reports from patient communities reveal a spectrum of approaches, from strict, meticulously documented regimens to more sporadic, trial-and-error use. Consistency in dosing, timing, and duration can affect not only the potential efficacy but also the risk of side effects or drug interactions. Missed doses, incorrect measurements, or premature discontinuation—often due to side effects, logistical challenges, or emotional distress—can all contribute to suboptimal outcomes. Conversely, overzealous dosing in hopes of accelerating results may increase risks without additional benefit.

The *quality and source of the product* introduces another layer of variability. Unlike pharmaceuticals dispensed through regulated channels, fenbendazole and ivermectin used in these protocols are often sourced from veterinary suppliers or online vendors, where standards for purity, potency, and labeling may not be consistent. Variations in formulation—powder, tablet, suspension—and the presence of excipients or contaminants can influence both absorption and safety. Some patients report marked differences in their experience after switching brands or batches, underscoring the importance of product consistency.

Co-administration with other therapies—whether conventional treatments like chemotherapy, targeted agents, or supportive supplements—further complicates the landscape. Drug-drug interactions can alter metabolism, increase toxicity, or reduce efficacy. For instance, both fenbendazole and ivermectin are metabolized by liver enzymes (notably CYP3A4), which are also involved in the processing of many oncology drugs. The addition of supplements such as curcumin, vitamin E, or CBD oil, as discussed in previous sections, may have synergistic or antagonistic effects, and these combinations are rarely studied systematically. The timing of administration relative to other treatments—before, during, or after cycles of chemotherapy—can also influence outcomes.

Monitoring and follow-up are essential yet often overlooked contributors to the diversity of reported experiences. Patients who engage in regular monitoring—through imaging, blood tests, or symptom diaries—are better positioned to detect subtle changes, adjust protocols, and communicate effectively with their healthcare team. In contrast, those who rely solely on subjective impressions may over- or underestimate the impact of the protocol. The absence of standardized endpoints makes it challenging to compare experiences or draw firm conclusions from anecdotal reports.

Finally, the *timeframe of observation* plays a decisive role. Some patients report rapid improvements in symptoms or tumor markers within weeks, while others see no change or experience delayed effects that only become apparent after months. The natural course of the disease, placebo responses, and fluctuations unrelated to the protocol can all influence perceptions of efficacy. Short-term benefits may not always translate into long-term outcomes, and vice versa.

In sum, the diversity of experiences with fenbendazole and ivermectin protocols reflects a tapestry woven from biological, practical, and contextual threads. Each factor—tumor type and genetics, disease stage, adherence, product quality, concurrent therapies, monitoring rigor, and timing—contributes to the final picture. Recognizing this complexity is not an argument against exploration, but rather a call for careful, critical assessment and open dialogue with healthcare professionals. By appreciating why experiences differ, patients and caregivers can approach these protocols with both curiosity and caution, maximizing the potential for benefit while minimizing risks.

6.5 Decision Triggers: When Patients Start, Pause, or Stop

In the context of reported fenbendazole and ivermectin protocols, the decision to start, pause, or stop these approaches is rarely straightforward. Patients and caregivers often navigate a complex landscape of clinical signals, logistical realities, and deeply personal considerations. A systematic approach to decision triggers is essential—not only to ensure safety and maximize potential benefit, but also to foster clear communication with the healthcare team. This verification checklist is designed to help readers recognize and document the multifaceted factors influencing these pivotal moments, providing a practical tool for reflection and discussion.

Establishing clear decision points can reduce uncertainty and support more confident, informed choices. By regularly reviewing clinical status, logistical feasibility, and personal readiness, patients and caregivers can better anticipate challenges and respond proactively to changes. This checklist does not replace clinical judgment or medical advice; rather, it serves as a structured prompt to ensure that no key consideration is overlooked, and that each decision is grounded in a holistic understanding of the current situation.

Decision Trigger Verification Checklist: Starting, Pausing, or Stopping Protocols

These items help ensure comprehensive assessment and quality control when considering changes to a reported protocol:

- **Clinical Stability and Baseline Assessment**

It is essential to verify the patient's current clinical status before initiating or modifying any protocol.

Check for recent lab results, imaging studies, and symptom assessments. Ensure there are no acute medical issues (e.g., infection, organ dysfunction) that would contraindicate starting or continuing the protocol.

- **Onset of New Symptoms or Adverse Effects**

Monitoring for new or worsening symptoms is critical to patient safety.

Document any changes in physical status (e.g., gastrointestinal distress, neurological symptoms, allergic reactions). Assess whether these symptoms may be related to the protocol or other underlying conditions.

- **Response to Conventional Therapies**

The relationship between reported protocols and ongoing standard treatments must be carefully considered.

Review recent oncology appointments, treatment cycles, and response evaluations. Consider whether starting, pausing, or stopping the protocol aligns with changes in the primary treatment plan.

- Drug Interactions and Contraindications

Potential interactions between fenbendazole, ivermectin, and other medications or supplements must be systematically reviewed.

Consult updated medication lists and cross-reference with known interaction profiles. Seek input from a pharmacist or oncologist as needed.

- Logistical Feasibility and Supply Chain

Access to reliable, high-quality sources of fenbendazole and ivermectin is a prerequisite for safe use.

Verify product authenticity, expiration dates, and ongoing availability. Consider potential disruptions (e.g., shipping delays, regulatory changes) that could necessitate pausing or stopping.

- Personal Readiness and Support Systems

Emotional, cognitive, and practical readiness are integral to protocol adherence and safety.

Assess the patient's understanding of the protocol, willingness to proceed, and availability of caregiver support. Evaluate whether stress, fatigue, or other personal factors may impact the ability to continue safely.

- Monitoring and Follow-up Plan

A clear plan for ongoing monitoring is essential for early detection of problems.

Ensure there is a schedule for symptom tracking, laboratory monitoring, and regular check-ins with the healthcare team. Confirm that mechanisms are in place for rapid response to adverse events.

- Alignment with Goals of Care

Decisions should always reflect the patient's overarching goals, values, and quality-of-life priorities.

Revisit advance directives, treatment preferences, and discussions about prognosis. Ensure that protocol use remains consistent with these goals.

USING THIS CHECKLIST:

- Review this checklist at each major decision point—before starting, during regular protocol use, and if considering a pause or discontinuation.
- Not all items will apply equally in every situation; adapt the checklist to individual circumstances while maintaining a comprehensive approach.
- If uncertainty arises regarding any item, prioritize open discussion with the treating oncologist or primary care provider.

QUALITY ASSURANCE:

- Thoroughly document each item, noting both positive findings and areas of uncertainty.
- Successful verification means that all relevant factors have been considered and that the decision—whether to start, pause, or stop—is made with full awareness of clinical, logistical, and personal dimensions.

A systematic approach to decision triggers not only enhances safety but also empowers patients and caregivers to participate actively in care decisions. By methodically verifying each element, the risk of oversights is minimized and the foundation for effective, collaborative care is strengthened. This process supports the ultimate goal: ensuring that every decision is as informed, intentional, and patient-centered as possible.

6.6 Integration with Conventional Treatment (Reported Approaches & Considerations)

Integrating reported use of fenbendazole and ivermectin with conventional cancer treatments is a process that demands careful planning, transparency, and ongoing communication. Patients and caregivers often approach this step with a mix of hope and apprehension—motivated by the desire for improved outcomes, yet aware of the complexities and uncertainties involved. Navigating this integration requires a structured approach that prioritizes safety, informed decision-making, and collaborative care.

Integrating Reported Protocols with Conventional Therapies

Overview: This process guides patients and caregivers through the essential steps for discussing, evaluating, and safely implementing reported fenbendazole and ivermectin protocols alongside chemotherapy, radiotherapy, immunotherapy, or other standard treatments.

Time Required: Several days to weeks (varies by case) | **Difficulty:** Moderate to Complex

What You'll Need:

- A detailed summary of your current cancer diagnosis, treatment plan, and medication list
- Reliable information on fenbendazole and ivermectin (including dosages, reported protocols, and potential interactions)
- A trusted oncologist or medical team willing to engage in open dialogue
- Tools for monitoring symptoms and side effects (e.g., symptom diary, lab results, digital apps)

Instructions:

Step 1: Prepare for the Conversation

- Gather all relevant medical records, including recent imaging, laboratory results, and a current list of prescribed and over-the-counter medications.
- Document your reasons for considering fenbendazole or ivermectin, referencing patient experiences or research summaries where appropriate.

• Prepare a list of specific questions and concerns for your oncologist.

• This preparation ensures your discussion is focused, evidence-based, and respectful of your clinician's expertise.

STEP 2: INITIATE AN OPEN DIALOGUE WITH YOUR MEDICAL TEAM

• Schedule a dedicated appointment to discuss integrative approaches. Clearly state your interest in reported fenbendazole or ivermectin protocols and share your research.

• Ask about potential interactions with your current treatments, and request their input on timing, dosing, and monitoring.

• Be transparent about any supplements or alternative therapies you are already using.

• Open communication helps build trust and allows your team to identify possible risks or contraindications early.

STEP 3: COMPREHENSIVE PRE-TREATMENT EVALUATION

• Undergo a thorough assessment, including baseline blood counts, liver and kidney function tests, and any other relevant parameters.

• Review your cancer's molecular profile, if available, as certain mutations or biomarkers may influence drug metabolism or response.

• Discuss your overall health status, comorbidities, and previous treatment-related side effects.

• This evaluation provides a clear starting point and helps anticipate potential complications.

STEP 4: STRATEGIC TIMING WITH CONVENTIONAL THERAPIES

• Coordinate the initiation of fenbendazole or ivermectin with your oncology team, considering the specific timing of chemotherapy, radiotherapy, or immunotherapy cycles.

• In some reported cases, patients have chosen to start these agents during treatment breaks or between cycles to minimize overlapping toxicities.

• For example, those receiving platinum-based chemotherapy have sometimes delayed fenbendazole initiation until blood counts recover.

• Timing is critical; improper overlap may increase the risk of side effects or reduce the efficacy of standard treatments.

STEP 5: INFORMED CONSENT AND DOCUMENTATION

• Ensure you fully understand the potential benefits, risks, and unknowns associated with off-label or non-standard use of these agents.

• Document your informed consent—ideally in writing—acknowledging that reported protocols are not standard of care and that data on safety and efficacy remain limited.

• Some patients choose to include family members or caregivers in these discussions to foster shared decision-making.

• Clear documentation protects both patient autonomy and the integrity of the clinical relationship.

STEP 6: ONGOING MONITORING AND SYMPTOM TRACKING

• Establish a regular schedule for clinical assessments and laboratory monitoring, tailored to your treatment regimen and risk factors.

• Use a symptom diary or digital health tool to record new or worsening symptoms, side effects, and any changes in quality of life.

• Promptly report concerning findings—such as jaundice, severe fatigue, or unexpected laboratory abnormalities—to your oncology team.

• Early detection of adverse events allows for timely intervention and may prevent serious complications.

STEP 7: PERIODIC REVIEW AND FOLLOW-UP

• Reassess the integration plan at each major treatment milestone (e.g., after each chemotherapy cycle, at imaging intervals, or during routine follow-up visits).

• Be prepared to adjust or discontinue fenbendazole or ivermectin if new evidence emerges, side effects develop, or if your cancer treatment plan changes.

• Regular follow-up ensures that your approach remains aligned with your evolving clinical situation and current best practices.

TROUBLESHOOTING:

- **Issue:** Oncologist is unfamiliar or uncomfortable with reported protocols → **Solution:** Provide peer-reviewed literature or case reports, seek a second opinion, or consult with a pharmacist experienced in integrative oncology.
- **Issue:** Unexpected side effects or lab abnormalities → **Solution:** Pause the non-standard agent, inform your medical team immediately, and undergo additional evaluation before resuming.
- **Issue:** Difficulty tracking symptoms or adherence → **Solution:** Use digital health tools, involve a caregiver, or request more frequent check-ins with your care team.

NEXT STEPS:

After completing these steps, continue to engage in open, honest communication with your medical team. Stay informed about new research and patient experiences, and revisit your integration plan as your treatment journey progresses. Remember, the landscape of integrative oncology is dynamic; flexibility and vigilance are essential.

Integrating reported fenbendazole and ivermectin protocols with conventional cancer treatments is not a one-time event but an ongoing process. It requires a balance of hope, caution, and collaboration. By following a structured approach, patients and caregivers can participate actively in their care, reduce uncertainty, and contribute to a safer, more informed treatment experience. This methodical integration, grounded in transparency and clinical oversight, is essential for those seeking to navigate the intersection of conventional and emerging therapies.

CHAPTER 7: SUPPLEMENTS AND SUPPORTIVE MEASURES

7.1 POPULAR ADD-ONS IN PATIENT REPORTS

In the context of reported off-label protocols involving fenbendazole and ivermectin, patients and caregivers frequently explore a range of supplementary substances—commonly referred to as "add-ons"—with the aim of enhancing efficacy, supporting general health, or mitigating side effects. The landscape of these add-ons is shaped by a blend of anecdotal experience, preliminary research, and, in some cases, established scientific rationale. However, the integration of additional supplements introduces complexity: potential interactions, cumulative toxicity, and the risk of inadvertently undermining conventional therapies. For these reasons, a systematic, evidence-informed approach to evaluating and selecting such add-ons is essential.

A well-constructed verification checklist serves as an indispensable tool for patients and caregivers navigating this terrain. It provides a structured method to assess the rationale, supporting evidence, dosing, safety profile, and practical criteria for each supplement under consideration. By working through this checklist, individuals can make more informed decisions, identify red flags early, and facilitate more productive discussions with healthcare professionals. This approach not only reduces uncertainty but also empowers patients to participate actively and responsibly in their care.

CHECKLIST FOR EVALUATING POPULAR ADD-ONS IN PATIENT REPORTS

These items help ensure comprehensive assessment and safe integration of supplements or substances frequently reported alongside fenbendazole and ivermectin protocols:

- **Name and Nature of Add-On**

Clear identification is fundamental to avoid confusion between substances with similar names or purposes.

Verify the exact supplement, its active ingredients, and formulation (e.g., curcumin vs. turmeric extract; vitamin D3 vs. D2).

- **Rationale for Use**

Understanding the underlying logic helps distinguish between evidence-based choices and speculative or anecdotal trends.

Check whether the supplement is intended for immune support, potential synergistic effects, side effect mitigation, or other specific goals.

- **Available Evidence**

The strength and quality of supporting data directly influence the risk-benefit calculation.

Review peer-reviewed studies, clinical trials, or case reports relevant to cancer settings. Note whether evidence is preclinical (cell/animal), observational, or from controlled human studies.

- **Typical Publicly Reported Dosing**

Accurate dosing is critical to avoid under- or overdosing, which can compromise safety and efficacy.

Identify commonly used doses from published reports, patient forums, or integrative oncology literature. Note the form (capsule, powder, liquid) and frequency.

- **Known Risks and Interactions**

Potential adverse effects and drug-supplement interactions must be proactively managed.

Screen for contraindications, known toxicities (e.g., liver or kidney effects), and documented interactions with chemotherapy, immunotherapy, or other medications.

- **Criteria for Selection**

Not every add-on is appropriate for every patient; individualized assessment is key.

Consider comorbidities, concurrent medications, allergies, and overall treatment goals. Evaluate whether the supplement aligns with the patient's clinical context and preferences.

- **Warning Signs and Criteria for Discontinuation**

Early detection of adverse effects or lack of benefit can prevent harm and optimize outcomes.

Establish clear parameters for when to pause or stop the supplement (e.g., new symptoms, lab abnormalities, allergic reactions, or guidance from a healthcare provider).

USING THIS CHECKLIST:

- Apply the checklist before introducing any new supplement or supportive measure, and revisit it periodically as circumstances change.

- Not all items will be relevant in every case; adapt the checklist to the patient's unique situation and priorities.
- If an item is not applicable, document the reason and move to the next consideration.

QUALITY ASSURANCE:

- Ensure each item is addressed thoroughly, drawing on reputable sources and, where possible, input from healthcare professionals.
- Successful verification means that no critical aspect—such as potential interactions or warning signs—has been overlooked, and that decisions are grounded in both evidence and individual context.

A disciplined, checklist-driven approach does not eliminate uncertainty, but it significantly reduces the likelihood of preventable errors and oversights. By systematically evaluating each potential add-on, patients and caregivers can approach integrative strategies with greater confidence, clarity, and safety—an essential foundation for navigating the complexities of supportive care in oncology.

7.2 Lifestyle and Nutrition Choices Patients Mention

Among patients navigating complex cancer protocols, lifestyle and nutrition choices frequently emerge as central themes in their personal strategies. These decisions are often described not only as adjuncts to pharmacological interventions but as pillars that support resilience, well-being, and a sense of agency during a time of profound uncertainty. While the diversity of reported approaches is considerable, several patterns and rationales recur in patient narratives, reflecting both individual experimentation and the influence of broader trends in integrative oncology.

Dietary modifications are among the most commonly mentioned lifestyle adaptations. Many patients report adopting diets perceived as anti-inflammatory or supportive of immune function. The ketogenic diet, for example, is frequently cited, with patients referencing its potential to "starve" cancer cells by limiting glucose availability. While robust clinical evidence in oncology remains limited, the underlying rationale is rooted in the metabolic theory of cancer, which posits that certain tumors rely heavily on glucose metabolism. Patients who pursue this approach often describe a sense of empowerment, noting that dietary discipline provides a tangible way to participate actively in their care. Others gravitate toward plant-forward or Mediterranean-style diets, emphasizing whole foods, abundant vegetables, healthy fats, and reduced processed sugars. These choices are often motivated by a desire to reduce systemic inflammation and support overall vitality, and some patients report improvements in energy levels, digestive comfort, or mood.

Beyond specific diets, the role of *nutritional supplementation* is frequently discussed in conjunction with broader lifestyle changes. Patients commonly mention the use of vitamin D, omega-3 fatty acids, and antioxidants, often after consulting with integrative practitioners or referencing emerging studies. The intention is typically to address deficiencies, modulate inflammation, or support immune function. However, patients also express awareness of the need for caution, especially regarding potential interactions with conventional therapies. This underscores the importance of open dialogue with healthcare providers, a theme explored in depth in later chapters.

Physical activity, tailored to individual capacity, is another cornerstone in many patients' routines. Even modest, regular movement—such as daily walks, gentle yoga, or stretching—is often credited with improving mood, reducing fatigue, and fostering a sense of normalcy. Some patients recount that structured exercise programs, when feasible, help maintain muscle mass, support cardiovascular health, and provide a psychological buffer against the sense of passivity that can accompany prolonged treatment. The degree of activity varies widely, with some individuals able to sustain vigorous routines, while others adjust their expectations in response to treatment side effects or disease progression.

Stress management emerges as a critical, if sometimes overlooked, dimension of supportive care. Patients frequently mention the adoption of mindfulness practices, meditation, or breathing exercises as tools to navigate anxiety, insomnia, and the emotional turbulence of a cancer diagnosis. These practices are often described as essential for maintaining clarity and composure in the face of uncertainty. For some, spiritual or religious rituals provide similar grounding, while others turn to creative outlets or support groups for emotional sustenance. The reported impact of these interventions is highly individualized, but many patients describe a cumulative benefit—a gradual strengthening of inner resources that complements the physical aspects of their regimen.

Sleep hygiene and rest are also recurrent themes in patient accounts. Strategies such as maintaining a consistent sleep schedule, minimizing screen time before bed, and creating a restful environment are cited as important for recovery and resilience. Fatigue is a pervasive challenge in oncology, and patients often experiment with various approaches to optimize rest, reporting that even incremental improvements in sleep quality can translate into better coping and improved daily functioning.

In synthesizing these experiences, a few overarching insights emerge. First, patients consistently emphasize the importance of *personalization*—tailoring lifestyle and nutrition choices to their own needs, preferences, and responses. There is a widespread recognition that no single approach is universally effective, and that flexibility is essential as circumstances evolve. Second, many patients describe a profound psychological benefit from making proactive choices, regardless of the specific regimen. The act of researching, selecting, and adhering to a lifestyle plan is often experienced as a reclaiming of agency, a way to participate meaningfully in the healing process.

Finally, patients frequently underscore the value of integrating these lifestyle measures into a broader, collaborative care plan. Rather than viewing nutrition, exercise, or stress management as alternatives to medical treatment, most see them as complementary—tools to enhance quality of life, support physical resilience, and foster hope. The cumulative effect, as reported in patient narratives, is not only a potential improvement in physical well being but also a deeper sense of engagement and purpose throughout the cancer journey.

These reported experiences, while diverse and sometimes anecdotal, offer valuable perspectives for patients and caregivers seeking to navigate the intersection of conventional and integrative care. They highlight the importance of informed experimentation, ongoing self-assessment, and open communication with the healthcare team—principles that underpin the practical guidance found throughout this handbook.

7.3 Monitoring Health and Progress

Effective monitoring of health and progress is a cornerstone of any integrative cancer approach, particularly when exploring protocols that fall outside standard oncologic care. The process is not merely a matter of tracking numbers; it is about cultivating an ongoing, informed dialogue with one's own body and healthcare team. A structured, methodical approach to monitoring can help distinguish between expected fluctuations and clinically significant changes, offering both reassurance and early warning when adjustments may be needed.

A comprehensive monitoring checklist begins with the selection of *relevant laboratory tests*. For most patients, this includes routine blood counts (CBC), liver and kidney function panels, and—where appropriate—tumor markers specific to the cancer type. These should be scheduled at intervals determined in collaboration with the treating oncologist, often every two to four weeks in the context of active disease or protocol changes. In some cases, more frequent monitoring may be warranted, particularly if new supplements or medications are introduced. Imaging studies such as CT, MRI, or PET scans remain the gold standard for assessing disease status, but their frequency is typically dictated by the clinical scenario and should always be coordinated with the oncology team.

Vital signs and physical parameters are equally important. Regular measurement of weight, blood pressure, heart rate, and temperature can reveal subtle shifts that might otherwise go unnoticed. For patients with advanced disease or those at risk for cachexia, even small changes in weight or appetite warrant attention. Many find it helpful to record these values weekly, using a dedicated notebook or digital health app. This not only creates a clear record for review but also encourages a sense of active participation in care.

Symptom tracking forms the third pillar of effective monitoring. It is essential to document both the presence and intensity of symptoms such as pain, fatigue, nausea, neurological changes, and gastrointestinal disturbances. Patients often benefit from using a simple 0–10 scale to rate symptom severity, noting any new or worsening issues promptly. For example, a patient who notices increasing neuropathy after starting a new supplement should record the onset, progression, and any associated factors. This level of detail can be invaluable when discussing concerns with the healthcare team, enabling more precise identification of potential causes and timely interventions.

Beyond the physical, monitoring should include *psychological and cognitive well-being*. Changes in mood, memory, or sleep patterns can signal underlying issues—whether related to treatment, disease progression, or the emotional toll of a cancer diagnosis. Brief daily or weekly notes about mood and energy levels can help capture trends that might otherwise be overlooked. Caregivers, too, play a vital role in this process, often noticing subtle behavioral shifts before the patient is fully aware of them.

Frequency of review is best tailored to the individual situation. In the initial weeks of a new protocol, daily symptom tracking and weekly review of physical parameters are prudent. Laboratory tests and imaging should follow the schedule agreed upon with the oncology team. As stability is achieved, intervals may be extended, but any new symptom or unexpected change should prompt immediate reassessment.

The value of meticulous record-keeping cannot be overstated. Whether using a traditional paper log or a digital platform, consistency is key. Each entry should include the date, time, and any relevant contextual notes—for example, the timing of supplement administration or recent changes in medication. This allows for the identification of patterns and correlations that may not be apparent in isolated data points. For instance, a gradual rise in liver enzymes might coincide with the introduction of a new supplement, prompting a timely discussion about potential hepatotoxicity.

Regular review of these records with the healthcare team is essential. Bringing a concise summary to appointments—highlighting trends, concerns, and specific questions—facilitates more productive conversations and supports shared decision-making. It is important to approach these discussions with openness, recognizing that not all changes are necessarily related to the protocol. The goal is not to self-diagnose, but to provide the clinical team with the most accurate and comprehensive information possible.

In summary, a robust monitoring checklist for patients and caregivers exploring fenbendazole, ivermectin, or other integrative protocols should include: scheduled laboratory tests and imaging; regular measurement of vital signs and physical parameters; systematic tracking of symptoms and side effects; attention to psychological and cognitive health, and consistent, organized record-keeping. This approach not only enhances safety but also empowers patients to engage proactively with their care, fostering a partnership with the medical team that is grounded in clarity, accuracy, and mutual respect.

PART IV
SAFETY, COMMUNICATION, AND INTEGRATION

CHAPTER 8: SAFETY FIRST

8.1 REPORTED SIDE EFFECTS AND RISKS

When considering the reported use of fenbendazole and ivermectin in oncology, a clear understanding of potential side effects and risks is essential. While both compounds have established safety profiles in their original veterinary and antiparasitic contexts, their off-label application in humans—especially in the context of cancer—warrants careful scrutiny. The variability in dosing, duration, and individual patient factors further underscores the importance of vigilance. Recognizing and categorizing adverse effects by severity and frequency enables patients and caregivers to make informed decisions and respond promptly to warning signs.

COMMON AND MILDLY REPORTED SIDE EFFECTS

Most frequently, users of fenbendazole and ivermectin report mild gastrointestinal disturbances. For fenbendazole, nausea, abdominal discomfort, and occasional diarrhea are the most cited symptoms. These effects are generally self-limiting and resolve with dose adjustment or temporary discontinuation. Similarly, ivermectin may cause mild digestive upset, including nausea, loose stools, or a metallic taste. Some individuals experience transient headaches, fatigue, or mild dizziness, particularly during the initial days of use. These symptoms, while uncomfortable, rarely necessitate medical intervention and often diminish as the body acclimates.

MODERATE AND LESS COMMON REACTIONS

A subset of patients report more pronounced effects, particularly with higher doses or prolonged use. Fenbendazole has been associated, albeit rarely, with mild elevations in liver enzymes, reflecting hepatic stress. Periodic monitoring of liver function is prudent, especially for those with preexisting hepatic conditions or concurrent use of other hepatotoxic medications. Ivermectin, when used at higher-than-approved doses, may provoke skin rashes, pruritus, or swelling, particularly in individuals with underlying sensitivities or compromised immune status. Some patients describe transient visual disturbances—blurred vision or changes in color perception—though these are infrequent and typically reversible.

Serious and Rare Adverse Events

Though uncommon, certain adverse effects demand immediate attention. Both drugs, at excessive doses or in susceptible individuals, carry the risk of severe allergic reactions. Anaphylaxis—characterized by rapid-onset swelling, difficulty breathing, hives, and hypotension—requires urgent medical intervention. Neurological symptoms such as persistent confusion, seizures, or loss of consciousness, though exceedingly rare, have been reported in isolated cases, especially with ivermectin. Hepatic injury, manifesting as jaundice (yellowing of the skin or eyes), dark urine, or severe abdominal pain, signals the need for prompt evaluation. In the context of cancer, where patients may already be immunocompromised or on complex medication regimens, the threshold for seeking medical advice should be low.

Warning Signs: When to Seek Immediate Medical Attention

Certain symptoms should never be ignored. Sudden onset of difficulty breathing, swelling of the face or throat, severe rash, chest pain, palpitations, or neurological changes such as confusion or seizures are all red flags. Additionally, signs of liver dysfunction—unexplained fatigue, jaundice, dark urine, or persistent nausea—warrant urgent assessment. For patients undergoing chemotherapy or other immunosuppressive treatments, even mild fevers or signs of infection should prompt early communication with the healthcare team.

Individual Risk Factors and Drug Interactions

It is essential to recognize that patient-specific factors—such as age, liver or kidney function, concurrent medications, and underlying health conditions—can significantly influence both the likelihood and severity of side effects. Fenbendazole and ivermectin may interact with other medications metabolized by the liver, potentially altering their efficacy or toxicity. For example, combining these agents with certain antifungals, antibiotics, or anticonvulsants can increase the risk of adverse reactions. A thorough medication review and consultation with a knowledgeable healthcare provider are indispensable steps before initiating any off-label protocol.

Verification Checklist: Comprehensive Review of Reported Side Effects and Risks

A systematic approach to monitoring and verification is crucial for anyone considering or actively using fenbendazole or ivermectin in an oncology setting. The following checklist is designed to ensure that all relevant aspects of safety and risk are thoroughly evaluated and not overlooked.

Adverse Effect and Risk Monitoring Checklist

- Documented Baseline Health Status

Establishes a reference point for detecting changes or new symptoms.

Verify recent liver and kidney function tests; note any preexisting conditions.

- Awareness of Common Side Effects

Prepares patient and caregiver for expected, typically mild reactions.

Review typical gastrointestinal, neurological, and dermatological symptoms.

- Recognition of Serious Warning Signs

Enables prompt response to potentially life-threatening events.

List symptoms requiring immediate medical attention (anaphylaxis, seizures, jaundice, severe rash, etc.).

- Review of Current Medications for Interactions

Reduces risk of compounded toxicity or reduced efficacy.

Cross-check all prescription, over-the-counter, and complementary medicines with a pharmacist or physician.

- Regular Monitoring Schedule Established

Facilitates early detection of emerging side effects or organ dysfunction.

Set intervals for laboratory testing (liver enzymes, kidney function) and clinical check-ins.

- Clear Communication Plan with Healthcare Team

Ensures rapid access to professional guidance if adverse effects arise.

Identify primary contact for urgent questions or symptom escalation.

- Documentation of All Symptoms and Changes

Supports accurate assessment and informed clinical decisions.

Maintain a daily log of physical and emotional changes, medication doses, and timing.

USING THIS CHECKLIST:

- Review before starting any new protocol and update regularly during use.
- Adapt items to individual circumstances—some may not apply to all patients.
- If a checklist item is not applicable, document the reason for clarity and future reference.

QUALITY ASSURANCE:

- Confirm that each item has been addressed and documented.
- Successful verification means both patient and caregiver understand potential risks, know what to monitor, and have a clear plan for escalation.

A systematic, checklist-driven approach provides reassurance and structure in what can otherwise be an uncertain process. By proactively identifying and monitoring for side effects and risks, patients and caregivers can participate more safely and confidently in their care journey, ensuring that no critical warning sign is missed and that interventions are timely and effective.

8.2 Possible Drug Interactions

In the context of integrative cancer care, the question of drug interactions acquires particular significance. Many patients already manage complex medication regimens, often involving chemotherapeutic agents, targeted therapies, immunomodulators, and supportive pharmaceuticals. The introduction of additional agents such as fenbendazole or ivermectin—originally developed for veterinary or antiparasitic use—demands a rigorous evaluation of potential pharmacological interactions. Even when these agents are considered "off-label" or experimental, their impact on metabolic pathways, drug transporters, and organ systems cannot be underestimated.

Both fenbendazole and ivermectin have demonstrated interactions with the cytochrome P450 enzyme system, a key player in drug metabolism. This system is responsible for the breakdown and clearance of a vast array of medications, including many commonly used in oncology. For example, fenbendazole is known to induce certain CYP enzymes, while ivermectin can act as both a substrate and inhibitor of CYP3A4. Such interactions may alter the plasma levels of co-administered drugs, potentially reducing efficacy or increasing toxicity. The risk is not limited to anticancer agents; medications for pain management, anticoagulation, infection prophylaxis, and even over-the-counter supplements may be affected.

The clinical implications are far from theoretical. Consider a patient on warfarin for venous thromboembolism prophylaxis—a scenario not uncommon in advanced cancer. The introduction of a CYP-modulating agent could shift warfarin metabolism, leading to subtherapeutic anticoagulation or, conversely, a dangerous elevation in bleeding risk. Similarly, interactions with certain azole antifungals, macrolide antibiotics, or antiepileptics may precipitate clinically significant changes in drug exposure. Even herbal supplements and nutraceuticals, frequently used by patients seeking integrative approaches, can further complicate the landscape.

Given this complexity, systematic verification of potential drug interactions is not merely a precaution—it is an essential component of safe, patient-centered care. The following checklist is designed to guide patients, caregivers, and clinicians through a structured evaluation of possible interactions when considering fenbendazole and ivermectin. It supports a thorough, stepwise approach, ensuring that no critical detail is overlooked in the pursuit of optimal safety.

DRUG INTERACTION VERIFICATION CHECKLIST

These items help ensure comprehensive coverage and quality control:

- **Review all current medications, including prescription, over-the-counter, and supplements**

Why this item is important to check: Drug interactions can arise from any substance with pharmacological activity, not just prescription medications.

What to look for or verify: Compile an up-to-date list of all substances being taken, including dosages and schedules.

- **Identify medications metabolized by cytochrome P450 enzymes, especially CYP3A4, CYP2C9, and CYP2D6**

Why this item is important to check: Fenbendazole and ivermectin can modulate these enzymes, affecting the metabolism of many drugs.

What to look for or verify: Cross-reference each medication with known CYP pathways; consult authoritative drug interaction resources or a clinical pharmacist.

- **Screen for high-risk drug classes: anticoagulants, immunosuppressants, anticonvulsants, antifungals, and chemotherapeutics**

Why this item is important to check: These classes are particularly susceptible to interactions that may have serious clinical consequences.

What to look for or verify: Note any drugs in these categories and flag for further review with a healthcare provider.

- **Assess for overlapping toxicities or organ system effects**

Why this item is important to check: Additive or synergistic toxicities (e.g., hepatotoxicity, neurotoxicity) may not be apparent without systematic review.

What to look for or verify: Compare known adverse effects of all agents for potential overlap; monitor for early signs of toxicity.

- **Consult with a physician or clinical pharmacist before initiating fenbendazole or ivermectin**

Why this item is important to check: Professional input is critical for evaluating complex interactions and making informed decisions.

What to look for or verify: Ensure that all planned changes are discussed and documented in the patient's medical record.

- Establish a monitoring plan for new or worsening symptoms after starting the protocol

Why this item is important to check: Early detection of adverse interactions can prevent escalation to serious harm.

What to look for or verify: Define specific symptoms to watch for, set a schedule for follow-up, and know when to seek urgent care.

USING THIS CHECKLIST:

- Use this checklist before introducing fenbendazole or ivermectin, and revisit it whenever there are changes to the medication regimen.
- The checklist is adaptable; not all items will apply to every patient, but each should be considered carefully.
- If a particular item is not relevant, document the rationale for exclusion and proceed to the next.

QUALITY ASSURANCE:

- Comprehensive checking involves collaboration between patient, caregiver, and healthcare professionals.
- Successful verification is achieved when all items are addressed, potential interactions are identified, and a clear plan is in place for monitoring and response.

Systematic checking of potential drug interactions is a cornerstone of safe integrative oncology practice. By following a structured approach, patients and caregivers can reduce uncertainty, anticipate challenges, and foster more informed, productive conversations with their healthcare team. This diligence not only safeguards against avoidable harm but also strengthens the foundation for collaborative, patient-centered care throughout the cancer journey.

8.3 Quality and Sourcing Considerations

Ensuring the quality and provenance of any product intended for personal use is a fundamental aspect of safety, but this becomes especially critical when considering substances outside standard pharmaceutical channels. For patients and caregivers exploring reported uses of fenbendazole or ivermectin, the risk of encountering substandard, counterfeit, or improperly stored products is significant. A systematic approach to evaluating quality and sourcing is therefore not just prudent—it is essential to minimize avoidable risks and to maintain the highest possible standards of safety.

A carefully constructed checklist can serve as a reliable safeguard, helping you navigate the complexities of product selection with greater confidence. By methodically verifying each aspect of a product's origin, handling, and presentation, you can reduce the likelihood of contamination, degradation, or mislabeling—issues that can have serious consequences, especially for individuals with compromised health. This checklist is designed to be comprehensive yet practical, guiding you through the critical elements that should be assessed before any product is considered for use.

Product Quality and Sourcing Verification Checklist

These items help ensure comprehensive coverage and quality control:

- **Manufacturer Verification**

Why this matters: The reputation and reliability of the manufacturer are foundational to product safety. Established manufacturers are more likely to adhere to rigorous quality standards and regulatory requirements.

What to check: Confirm the manufacturer's full name, location, and, if possible, their registration or certification status. Look for products made by companies with a documented track record in veterinary or pharmaceutical production.

- **Certification and Regulatory Compliance**

Why this matters: Certifications (such as GMP—Good Manufacturing Practice—or ISO standards) indicate adherence to recognized quality and safety protocols.

What to check: Examine the packaging and product documentation for official seals, batch numbers, and certification marks. Verify these details through the manufacturer's website or regulatory databases where possible.

- Packaging Integrity

Why this matters: Intact, undamaged packaging helps ensure that the product has not been tampered with or exposed to environmental factors that could compromise its quality.

What to check: Inspect for unbroken seals, clear labeling, and absence of tears, punctures, or discoloration. Packaging should include lot numbers and expiration dates, printed clearly and consistently.

- Expiration Date and Batch Information

Why this matters: Using expired or improperly labeled products can result in reduced efficacy or increased risk of adverse effects.

What to check: Confirm that the expiration date is current and that batch or lot numbers are present. Avoid products with missing, altered, or illegible dates.

- Trusted Source of Purchase

Why this matters: Reliable distribution channels reduce the risk of counterfeit or mishandled products entering the supply chain.

What to check: Purchase only from reputable pharmacies, veterinary suppliers, or authorized distributors. Be wary of online marketplaces or private sellers without verifiable credentials or customer support.

- Product Documentation and Information

Why this matters: Comprehensive documentation supports transparency and traceability, which are essential for safety and accountability.

What to check: Look for accompanying product inserts, safety data sheets, and clear usage instructions. Documentation should match the product and be free of translation errors or inconsistencies.

QUALITY ASSURANCE:

• Take time to review each item thoroughly—do not rely solely on first impressions or seller assurances.

• Successful verification means every item is clearly addressed, with supporting evidence where possible (such as photographs, receipts, or documentation from the supplier).

• When in doubt, err on the side of caution and consult with a healthcare professional or pharmacist before proceeding.

A systematic approach to quality and sourcing is not merely a bureaucratic exercise—it is a critical layer of protection for both patients and caregivers. By making these checks routine, you reinforce a culture of safety, reduce the risk of preventable harm, and support informed, confident decision-making throughout your care journey.

8.4 Contraindications & Special Populations

Contraindications and the identification of special populations are critical components of safe protocol consideration, especially when exploring off-label or adjunctive therapies such as fenbendazole and ivermectin. While these agents have generated interest due to emerging preclinical and anecdotal reports, their use outside established indications demands heightened vigilance. Not every patient is an appropriate candidate, and the risks can be significant if underlying factors are overlooked.

Pregnancy represents a clear contraindication for both fenbendazole and ivermectin. The available data, primarily from animal studies and veterinary use, indicate potential teratogenicity and embryotoxicity, particularly with fenbendazole at high doses. Ivermectin, likewise, has demonstrated adverse fetal effects in animal models, and its safety profile in human pregnancy remains insufficiently characterized. For these reasons, both agents are categorically avoided in pregnant individuals. The potential risks to fetal development far outweigh any theoretical benefit, and no reputable guidelines support their use in this population. For women of childbearing potential, effective contraception is essential during and after any experimental use, and pregnancy testing should precede consideration of these agents.

Children and adolescents constitute another vulnerable group. The pharmacokinetics and pharmacodynamics of fenbendazole and ivermectin are not fully defined in pediatric oncology, and dosing regimens established for parasitic infections may not translate safely to oncologic contexts. Children's developing organ systems, particularly the liver and kidneys, may be less able to metabolize or excrete these drugs, increasing the risk of toxicity. Moreover, the long-term effects of off-label use in this population are unknown. For these reasons, the use of fenbendazole or ivermectin in pediatric cancer patients should be approached with extreme caution, if at all, and always under direct supervision of a pediatric oncologist familiar with investigational therapies.

Underlying hepatic or renal impairment is a further contraindication that must not be underestimated. Both fenbendazole and ivermectin undergo hepatic metabolism and are excreted, at least in part, via the biliary and renal systems.

In patients with compromised liver or kidney function—whether due to cancer involvement, prior chemotherapy, or comorbid conditions—drug clearance may be significantly reduced. This can result in accumulation of the active compound or its metabolites, heightening the risk of adverse effects such as hepatotoxicity, neurotoxicity, or systemic toxicity. Clinical experience in these populations is extremely limited, and there are no established dose adjustments or monitoring protocols for off-label oncologic use. Baseline and ongoing assessment of liver and kidney function is essential if these agents are being considered, and even then, the threshold for withholding or discontinuing therapy should be low.

Immunocompromised patients, including those with advanced malignancies or on immunosuppressive therapy, represent another special population requiring careful consideration. While fenbendazole and ivermectin are not inherently immunosuppressive, their impact on immune function in the context of cancer and its treatment is not fully understood. There is also the potential for atypical infections or altered drug metabolism in this group, further complicating risk assessment. The possibility of drug-drug interactions is heightened, as immunocompromised patients are often prescribed multiple medications with narrow therapeutic windows.

Patients with a history of hypersensitivity or allergic reactions to benzimidazole compounds (for fenbendazole) or to avermectins (for ivermectin) are absolutely contraindicated. Even mild prior reactions can escalate with repeated exposure, and anaphylaxis, although rare, has been documented in both veterinary and human contexts. A thorough allergy history is indispensable before any consideration of these protocols.

Beyond these primary categories, it is important to recognize that **individual variability**—including genetic differences in drug metabolism, nutritional status, and concurrent illnesses—can profoundly influence both efficacy and safety. For example, certain populations may carry polymorphisms in cytochrome P450 enzymes or P-glycoprotein transporters, altering drug levels unpredictably. While routine genetic screening is not standard practice, awareness of these factors underscores the need for individualized assessment and close monitoring.

Clinical supervision is not a formality but a necessity. The potential for adverse outcomes increases dramatically when protocols are self-administered without medical oversight. Only a healthcare professional can adequately assess the interplay of comorbidities, concurrent medications, and evolving clinical status. Moreover, the subtle onset of toxicity—such as mild elevations in liver enzymes or early neurological symptoms—may be missed without regular laboratory and clinical evaluation.

In summary, while the search for new therapeutic avenues is both understandable and commendable, it must be grounded in a clear-eyed appraisal of risk. **Pregnancy, pediatric age, hepatic or renal impairment, immunocompromised status, and known hypersensitivity** are all strong contraindications or require heightened caution. The importance of medical supervision cannot be overstated; it is the cornerstone of safe and responsible exploration of any integrative or adjunctive protocol. As with all aspects of cancer care, the principle of "first, do no harm" must remain paramount, guiding both patients and caregivers in their decision-making.

8.5 Regulatory & Ethical Context (Off-Label Use)

The use of fenbendazole and ivermectin in oncology is situated within a complex regulatory and ethical landscape, shaped by evolving scientific evidence, patient advocacy, and the boundaries of medical law. At the heart of this landscape lies the concept of *off-label* use—prescribing a medication for an indication, dosage, or patient population not explicitly approved by regulatory authorities such as the U.S. Food and Drug Administration (FDA) or the European Medicines Agency (EMA). Understanding the nuances of this practice is essential for patients and caregivers navigating unconventional treatment paths.

Off-label use is both common and legally permissible in many countries, especially in oncology, where therapeutic innovation often outpaces formal regulatory approval. In the United States, the FDA regulates the approval and marketing of drugs, but once a drug is approved for one indication, licensed physicians may prescribe it for other uses based on their clinical judgment. This flexibility is crucial in cancer care, where new evidence or urgent need may justify trying therapies outside their original scope. However, this freedom is balanced by professional and ethical obligations: physicians must base their decisions on the best available evidence, prioritize patient safety, and ensure informed consent.

The EMA, which oversees drug regulation across the European Union, operates under similar principles. While the agency authorizes drugs for specific indications, it does not restrict physicians from prescribing them off-label when medically justified. National laws and medical codes of conduct further guide these practices, often requiring that off-label use be supported by scientific rationale, documented in the patient's medical record, and discussed transparently with the patient. In some European countries, reimbursement for off-label treatments may be restricted, adding another layer of complexity for patients seeking access to these protocols.

Globally, the regulatory environment varies considerably. In Canada and Australia, for example, off-label prescribing is permitted but subject to oversight by professional colleges and, at times, additional documentation or justification. In other jurisdictions, the legal framework may be less clear, and patients may encounter significant barriers to obtaining non-standard therapies. It is not uncommon for individuals to source medications independently, particularly when conventional options have been exhausted, but this approach carries legal and safety risks, including the potential for counterfeit or substandard products.

Ethical considerations are inseparable from the regulatory context. Physicians are entrusted with the responsibility to act in their patients' best interests, which includes weighing the potential benefits of off-label treatments against the risks and uncertainties. The principle of *informed consent* is paramount: patients must be fully apprised of the evidence supporting the use of fenbendazole or ivermectin, the limitations of current knowledge, and the possible side effects or interactions. In practice, this means a candid conversation about what is known, what remains uncertain, and how the decision aligns with the patient's goals and values.

Healthcare teams must also be mindful of the broader implications of off-label use. While patient autonomy is a core value, clinicians cannot ethically offer treatments that lack a reasonable scientific basis or that might expose patients to undue harm. The line between compassionate use and experimental therapy can be thin, particularly when hope is a powerful motivator and information is rapidly disseminated online. This underscores the importance of grounding decisions in credible data, as discussed in Chapters 3, 4, and 5, and maintaining open, ongoing dialogue with the patient and their support network.

Practical challenges often arise when integrating off-label protocols into care. Insurance coverage is a recurrent issue; many insurers will not reimburse medications used outside of approved indications, leaving patients to bear the financial burden. Hospitals and pharmacies may have policies restricting the dispensing of drugs for non-standard uses, and some clinicians may be reluctant to participate in protocols they perceive as lacking sufficient evidence or regulatory support. These barriers can be discouraging, but understanding the regulatory framework empowers patients and caregivers to ask informed questions and advocate for their needs within established legal and ethical boundaries.

Ultimately, the decision to pursue off-label use of fenbendazole or ivermectin should be made collaboratively, with the guidance of a knowledgeable healthcare team. Documenting the rationale for treatment, monitoring outcomes closely, and remaining vigilant for new evidence or safety signals are all essential practices. As research continues to evolve, the regulatory and ethical landscape may shift, potentially opening new avenues—or imposing new constraints—on the use of these and other repurposed drugs in oncology.

For those considering or already engaged in off-label protocols, staying informed about local regulations, maintaining transparent communication with healthcare providers, and grounding decisions in both scientific evidence and personal values are the cornerstones of responsible, ethical care. This approach not only supports individual well-being but also contributes to a broader culture of safety, integrity, and progress in cancer treatment.

CHAPTER 9: TALKING WITH YOUR HEALTHCARE TEAM

9.1 HOW TO START THE CONVERSATION

Initiating a conversation with your healthcare team about the reported use of fenbendazole or ivermectin in an oncological context requires both preparation and sensitivity. Medical professionals are trained to base their recommendations on established evidence, and new or unconventional approaches may be met with caution. However, clear and respectful communication can open a constructive dialogue that supports shared decision-making and ensures your care remains safe and coordinated.

Begin by framing your intentions transparently. Physicians appreciate when patients are proactive and well-informed, but it is equally important to convey that your interest in these protocols comes from a desire to understand all possible options, not from a place of distrust. For example, you might say, "I've been reading about some alternative protocols, specifically involving fenbendazole and ivermectin, and I'd like to discuss what is known about their use in cancer care." This approach signals that you value your doctor's expertise and want their perspective, rather than presenting a decision already made.

It is helpful to express your reasoning and goals. You might add, "I'm interested in learning whether these approaches could complement my current treatment, and I want to make sure anything I consider is safe and does not interfere with my ongoing therapies." This reassures your physician that you are not seeking to abandon evidence-based care, but to explore adjunctive possibilities with professional guidance.

Asking open-ended questions can foster a more collaborative atmosphere. Consider phrasing such as, "What have you heard about these protocols in oncology?" or "Are there any known risks or interactions with my current treatment?" These questions invite your healthcare provider to share their knowledge and concerns, and they demonstrate that you are seeking a balanced, informed discussion. If you sense hesitation or unfamiliarity, it is appropriate to ask, "Would you be willing to look into the latest research with me, or refer me to someone who might have more experience with these agents?" This acknowledges the limits of current knowledge while emphasizing your commitment to safety.

Bringing supporting materials can be valuable, but choose reputable sources—peer-reviewed studies, clinical guidelines, or summaries from respected institutions. Present these resources as a basis for discussion rather than as evidence to persuade. For example: "I found a few recent studies on this topic; could we review them together to understand the potential benefits and risks?" This positions your doctor as a partner in evaluating the information rather than an adversary.

It is also wise to anticipate concerns about safety, drug interactions, and the lack of regulatory approval for these uses. You might preemptively address this by stating, "I understand that these medications are not approved for cancer treatment, and I want to be cautious. My goal is to make informed decisions and avoid anything that could be harmful or interfere with my care." This demonstrates your commitment to responsible decision-making and helps reduce defensiveness.

If you feel nervous or unsure, consider rehearsing the conversation or bringing a caregiver or advocate to the appointment. Sometimes, having another person present can help clarify your intentions and ensure that key points are addressed. You might say, "I've asked my caregiver to join us today because we both want to make sure we understand all aspects of my treatment options."

Throughout the discussion, remain open to feedback and willing to adjust your expectations. Not all clinicians will be familiar with these protocols, and some may express skepticism. If that occurs, listen carefully, ask for clarification, and request specific reasons for any recommendations or cautions. For example: "Can you help me understand your concerns about these medications? Are there particular risks I should be aware of?" This invites a more nuanced exchange and may uncover considerations you had not previously recognized.

Ultimately, the objective is to foster an environment of mutual respect and trust. By approaching the conversation with curiosity, transparency, and a willingness to listen, you enable your healthcare team to support you more effectively—whether that means helping you evaluate new information, monitoring for potential side effects, or simply acknowledging your need to explore every avenue. In this way, you remain an active participant in your care, guided by both scientific evidence and open communication.

9.2 Finding Supportive Practitioners

Identifying practitioners who are open to integrative approaches requires both discernment and a structured strategy. In the context of cancer care, where conventional protocols dominate and skepticism toward unconventional therapies can be high, finding a supportive professional is not simply a matter of searching for a title. It involves evaluating a practitioner's openness, expertise, and ethical standards with care.

The first step is to clarify what "supportive" means in your specific context. For some, it may be a physician willing to discuss the evidence behind off-label or repurposed drugs like fenbendazole and ivermectin. For others, it could involve a multidisciplinary team—oncologists, integrative medicine specialists, pharmacists, and nurses—who collaborate to ensure safety while respecting patient autonomy. The ideal practitioner demonstrates a balance of scientific rigor and respectful curiosity, neither dismissing unconventional ideas outright nor endorsing them without scrutiny.

A practical approach begins with targeted research. Professional directories from reputable organizations such as the Society for Integrative Oncology (SIO), the Academic Consortium for Integrative Medicine & Health, or national medical boards can be invaluable starting points. These platforms often list practitioners who have formal training in integrative or complementary medicine and adhere to established ethical guidelines. Hospital-based integrative oncology programs, frequently affiliated with major cancer centers, provide another layer of credibility. When reviewing practitioner profiles, look for evidence of continuing education in integrative therapies, published research, or participation in multidisciplinary tumor boards—these are strong indicators of genuine engagement with evolving science.

Patient advocacy groups and peer networks also serve as critical resources. Communities such as Inspire, Cancer Support Community, or disease-specific forums often share firsthand experiences and recommendations. While anecdotal, these insights can reveal which practitioners are known for thoughtful dialogue and patient-centered care. However, always cross-reference such recommendations with formal credentials and professional standing.

Evaluating a practitioner's reliability involves more than checking degrees or affiliations. During initial consultations, pay attention to how the practitioner responds to your questions about integrative protocols. A reliable professional will acknowledge the current limitations of evidence, discuss potential risks and interactions, and emphasize the importance of monitoring and communication with your entire care team. They will not promise cures or downplay the seriousness of off-label drug use. Instead, they will offer a nuanced perspective, perhaps suggesting ways to track side effects, coordinate lab monitoring, or facilitate open communication with your primary oncologist.

Transparency is another hallmark of trustworthy practitioners. They should be willing to explain their reasoning, share relevant research, and outline the boundaries of their expertise. For example, an integrative oncologist might clarify that while preclinical data on fenbendazole is intriguing, robust clinical trials are lacking, and any use should be approached with caution. They may also provide guidance on how to document and report any adverse effects, ensuring that your care remains coordinated and safe.

Red flags are equally important to recognize. Be wary of practitioners who discourage communication with your primary oncology team, require large upfront payments, or make sweeping claims about unproven therapies. The absence of informed consent, reluctance to discuss potential drug interactions, or lack of transparency about their own experience with integrative protocols should prompt caution. Reliable professionals will always prioritize patient safety, evidence-based practice, and shared decision-making.

In practice, many patients find that the most supportive practitioners are those who see themselves as partners in care. They respect your right to explore complementary options and help you do so as safely as possible. They are willing to consult the latest literature, reach out to colleagues for second opinions, and adapt their recommendations as new data emerge. This collaborative spirit is particularly valuable when navigating areas of uncertainty, such as the reported use of fenbendazole or ivermectin in cancer care.

Ultimately, the process of finding a supportive practitioner is iterative. It may involve several consultations, ongoing dialogue, and a willingness to seek second opinions. By combining careful research, critical evaluation, and open communication, you can build a team that not only acknowledges your values but also upholds the highest standards of professional integrity. In the evolving landscape of integrative oncology, such partnerships are essential for informed, empowered decision-making.

9.3 Navigating Disagreement

Disagreements between patients and healthcare teams are not uncommon, especially when considering integrative or off-label approaches such as those discussed in this book. The clinical environment is shaped by evidence-based protocols, regulatory frameworks, and the collective experience of medical professionals, while patients and caregivers often bring a unique urgency, lived experience, and a desire to explore every possible avenue. Navigating these differences requires both clarity and respect, as well as a practical strategy for ensuring that your voice is heard and your concerns are addressed constructively.

The first step in managing disagreement is to approach the conversation as a partnership, not a confrontation. Physicians and nurses are trained to prioritize patient safety and adhere to established standards of care. When presenting your interest in protocols involving fenbendazole or ivermectin, framing your questions in terms of curiosity and shared problem-solving can foster a more open dialogue. For example, you might say, "I've come across some patient-reported protocols and emerging research on these compounds. Can we discuss the potential risks and benefits together?" This approach signals your respect for their expertise while asserting your right to participate in decisions about your care.

It is essential to listen carefully to the rationale behind your healthcare team's concerns. Medical professionals may express reservations based on the current evidence base, regulatory status, or potential for drug interactions. Rather than viewing these objections as barriers, consider them as valuable information that can help you make more informed choices. If a clinician is particularly resistant, ask for clarification: "Could you help me understand your main concerns? Are there specific risks you're worried about in my case?" This not only demonstrates your willingness to engage thoughtfully but can also reveal areas where additional information or compromise may be possible.

Documentation is a powerful tool in these situations. After each discussion, summarize the main points, questions raised, and any decisions or next steps agreed upon. This can be as simple as a dated note in a dedicated notebook or a brief email sent to your provider, recapping your understanding of the conversation. For example: "Following our discussion today, I understand that you have concerns about potential liver toxicity with fenbendazole. I appreciate your suggestion to monitor liver function tests if I proceed. I will keep you informed about any changes." This practice not only creates a clear record but also reinforces your commitment to transparency and shared responsibility.

If disagreement persists, consider requesting a multidisciplinary meeting or a second opinion within the same institution. Many cancer centers have tumor boards or integrative medicine specialists who can offer additional perspectives. Bringing another professional into the conversation may help bridge gaps in understanding or validate your concerns in a different context. It is also appropriate to ask about the process for documenting your wishes in the medical record, particularly if you intend to pursue an adjunctive protocol independently. Most healthcare systems have mechanisms for noting patient preferences and advance directives, ensuring that your choices are visible to all members of your care team.

Throughout these interactions, maintaining a tone of mutual respect is paramount. Express appreciation for your team's expertise and acknowledge the complexity of your situation. Avoid adversarial language or ultimatums, which can inadvertently close doors to future collaboration. Instead, focus on building a relationship grounded in trust, even when opinions diverge. Over time, this approach can foster a more flexible, patient-centered dynamic—one in which your values and priorities are recognized as integral to the decision-making process.

Ultimately, the goal is not to "win" an argument but to arrive at a plan that balances innovation with safety, hope with realism. By documenting discussions, seeking clarification, and engaging additional expertise when needed, you can navigate disagreement with professionalism and poise. This process not only protects your interests but also models the kind of collaborative care that is essential in complex, evolving fields such as integrative oncology.

PART V
PATIENT AND CAREGIVER STORIES

CHAPTER 10: PATIENT JOURNEYS

10.1 FROM DESPERATION TO DETERMINATION

In the landscape of cancer care, moments of profound uncertainty and fear often serve as the catalyst for transformation. For many patients, the journey toward integrative or alternative protocols begins not with optimism, but with the stark reality of limited options. The stories that follow are not tales of miraculous cures, but rather of individuals who, when confronted with daunting prognoses or diminishing returns from conventional therapies, found within themselves a renewed sense of agency. Their paths illustrate how desperation can evolve into determination, shaping a proactive approach to care that is both informed and intentional.

Consider the experience of a patient diagnosed with metastatic colorectal cancer after standard chemotherapy regimens had failed to halt disease progression. Facing a future measured in months, she encountered online patient forums discussing the off-label use of fenbendazole. Initially skeptical, she was struck by the volume of anecdotal reports and the measured tone of discussions—patients were not abandoning medical advice, but seeking to supplement it. What distinguished her journey was a methodical approach: she compiled published studies, documented every step, and maintained open communication with her oncologist. This diligence enabled her to monitor for adverse effects, adjust her protocol based on emerging evidence, and maintain a sense of control over her care. While her disease remained incurable, she reported improved symptom management and a restored sense of purpose, underscoring the psychological impact of feeling actively involved in her treatment decisions.

Another case involved a man with advanced non-small cell lung cancer, whose response to immunotherapy had plateaued. Motivated by a desire to leave no stone unturned, he began investigating the scientific literature on ivermectin's potential anticancer properties. What began as a late-night search soon became a structured inquiry: he analyzed preclinical studies, consulted with pharmacists about drug interactions, and joined patient-led support groups to exchange practical tips. His approach was characterized by a careful balancing of hope and realism—he was acutely aware of the limitations of current evidence, but equally unwilling to forgo a potentially beneficial adjunct. By integrating ivermectin into his regimen under close medical supervision, he was able to navigate side effects and maintain quality of life, while also contributing his observations to ongoing patient registries.

These narratives share several common threads. First, the transition from desperation to determination is rarely a linear process. It is shaped by moments of doubt, incremental learning, and the gradual accumulation of *practical knowledge*. Patients often describe a pivotal moment—a conversation with a caregiver, a new research article, or a supportive online community—that shifts their mindset from passive recipient to active participant. This shift is not merely psychological; it has tangible implications for protocol adherence, side effect monitoring, and communication with healthcare providers.

Second, the role of *information literacy* cannot be overstated. The patients who navigated these alternative or integrative paths most effectively were those who invested significant effort in understanding both the scientific rationale and the practical logistics of their chosen protocols. They scrutinized sources, distinguished between anecdote and evidence, and sought professional input whenever possible. This diligence not only reduced the risk of harm, but also empowered them to ask informed questions and advocate for their preferences within the medical system.

Caregivers, too, play a pivotal role in this transformation. In many cases, it is the caregiver who first encounters new research, organizes medication schedules, or provides the emotional support necessary to sustain motivation. Their involvement often marks the difference between an improvised experiment and a carefully managed adjunctive therapy. The collaborative dynamic that emerges—patient and caregiver as partners in exploration—serves as a foundation for resilience and adaptability.

It is important to acknowledge that these journeys are not universally successful, nor are they free from setbacks. Some patients encountered unanticipated side effects, logistical challenges in sourcing medications, or emotional fatigue from the relentless pursuit of new information. Yet, even in the face of these obstacles, the act of *engagement* itself was frequently cited as a source of hope. For many, the process of researching, planning, and executing a protocol—regardless of the ultimate outcome—restored a sense of agency that had been eroded by the unpredictability of cancer.

Ultimately, these stories illustrate a central truth: the movement from desperation to determination is not about rejecting conventional medicine, but about reclaiming a measure of control in an inherently uncertain context. By approaching alternative protocols with rigor, skepticism, and open communication, patients and caregivers can transform fear into purposeful action. Their experiences, while deeply personal, offer valuable insights for others navigating similar crossroads—reminding us that, even in the most challenging circumstances, informed determination can be a powerful force for both practical and psychological well-being.

10.2 Reported Improvements and Stable Cases

Across the landscape of patient-reported experiences with fenbendazole and ivermectin, a recurring theme emerges: individuals and their caregivers often describe periods of unexpected improvement or stabilization, particularly in cases where conventional options had been exhausted or had shown diminishing returns. While these accounts cannot substitute for controlled clinical data, they offer valuable insight into how these protocols are being applied in real-world settings and what outcomes have been observed.

One illustrative case involves a 62-year-old man with metastatic non-small cell lung cancer, refractory to multiple lines of chemotherapy and immunotherapy. After learning about the off-label use of fenbendazole through patient forums and preliminary research, he initiated a protocol consisting of 222 mg of fenbendazole daily, cycling five days on and two days off, in combination with his ongoing supportive care regimen. Over the subsequent three months, imaging revealed a halt in tumor progression, with some nodal lesions showing modest reduction in size. His oncologist, while cautious, noted the unexpected stability given the prior trajectory of disease. The patient reported improved energy and appetite, and these effects persisted for nearly eight months before further progression occurred. This case underscores the importance of context: the patient's stabilization coincided with the introduction of fenbendazole, but the multifactorial nature of cancer progression and response must always be considered.

Another frequently cited scenario involves patients with advanced colorectal cancer who have integrated ivermectin into their care plans. In one such case, a 54-year-old woman, previously treated with standard chemotherapy and targeted therapies, began self-administering ivermectin at a dose of 12 mg every other day. Over a six-month period, serial imaging demonstrated stable disease, and tumor markers remained unchanged. She maintained this regimen alongside vitamin D supplementation and careful nutritional monitoring, as outlined in Chapter 7. Notably, her quality of life metrics improved, with reduced fatigue and less gastrointestinal discomfort. While causality cannot be established, the temporal association between the introduction of ivermectin and disease stabilization was striking to both patient and care team, prompting ongoing observation and documentation.

It is also essential to highlight cases where reported improvements were not limited to imaging or laboratory results, but extended to subjective well-being and daily function. For example, several patients with glioblastoma—a notoriously aggressive brain tumor—have described periods of stabilization lasting four to six months after initiating fenbendazole, often in combination with other supportive measures such as curcumin, vitamin E, and intermittent fasting. In these instances, families noted improved cognitive clarity and reduced seizure frequency, contributing to a better overall quality of life. These effects, while not always mirrored by dramatic radiological changes, were meaningful to patients and caregivers alike.

A pattern emerges from these narratives: **reported improvements and stabilization most often occur in the context of integrative approaches**, where fenbendazole or ivermectin are added to existing supportive or palliative care regimens rather than used in isolation. Duration of benefit varies widely, with some individuals experiencing several months of stability, while others report more transient effects. Importantly, in nearly all cases, patients maintained close communication with their healthcare teams, as emphasized in Chapter 9, and used structured monitoring tools to track both objective and subjective outcomes.

The diversity of reported protocols—ranging from daily low-dose administration to intermittent cycles, and often accompanied by adjunctive supplements—reflects the experimental nature of this approach. It also highlights the need for individualized planning, careful observation, and ongoing dialogue with medical professionals. The stories collected here do not offer guarantees, but they do provide a nuanced perspective on what may be possible when patients and caregivers pursue informed, closely monitored experimentation within the boundaries of safety and ethical care.

In summary, while the evidence remains anecdotal and should be interpreted with caution, **these patient journeys illustrate the potential for periods of improvement or stabilization** in otherwise challenging oncologic scenarios. They also underscore the importance of context, comprehensive care, and critical self-monitoring. As research evolves, these lived experiences will continue to inform both clinical inquiry and patient decision making, offering hope tempered by realism and a commitment to evidence-based practice.

10.3 When It Didn't Work

Among the many patient journeys chronicled in this field, some stand out not for the breakthroughs they deliver, but for the sobering lessons they impart. While stories of improvement and stability often capture attention, it is equally important to examine those instances where reported use of fenbendazole or ivermectin did not yield the hoped-for results. These narratives, though difficult, offer critical insights into the complexities of cancer, the unpredictability of individual response, and the importance of maintaining a grounded perspective when evaluating integrative approaches.

One recurring theme in these accounts is the **diversity of patient backgrounds and disease trajectories**. For example, Maria, a 62-year-old with advanced ovarian cancer, began a self-directed protocol after exhausting standard therapies. Despite meticulous adherence to a widely shared regimen, she experienced no measurable tumor regression over several months. Her oncologist, kept fully informed, noted that her disease continued to progress at a rate consistent with its natural course. Maria's experience underscores a reality often echoed by clinicians: *not all tumors, nor all patients, respond in the same way to any intervention*, whether conventional or experimental.

In another case, Samuel, a 54-year-old diagnosed with metastatic colorectal cancer, incorporated fenbendazole alongside his prescribed chemotherapy. He reported no improvement in energy, pain, or tumor markers, and imaging revealed continued spread. Samuel and his family reflected that, while the protocol had been undertaken with hope and careful monitoring, it did not alter the clinical outcome. Importantly, Samuel's care team maintained open dialogue, ensuring that the addition of non-standard agents did not interfere with ongoing treatment or delay evidence-based decisions.

The reasons underlying lack of response are multifactorial and, in many cases, remain speculative. **Biological variability** plays a significant role. Genetic differences between tumors, variations in drug metabolism, and the unique interplay of immune factors can all influence outcomes. In some instances, patients began these protocols at very advanced stages, when disease burden and organ compromise limited the potential for any intervention—conventional or otherwise—to effect meaningful change. Others may have encountered issues with absorption, dosing inconsistencies, or unrecognized drug interactions that blunted any possible effect.

Several patients also reported that, despite initial anecdotal reports or online testimonials, their own experiences did not match the optimism found in some communities. For instance, Anna, who tried ivermectin after reading about its purported benefits, described a sense of frustration when her scans showed continued progression. She later reflected that, while disappointment was inevitable, the process of trying the protocol had at least given her a sense of agency at a time when options were few. Her story highlights a subtle but important lesson: *the psychological impact of hope and action can be meaningful, even when clinical benefit is not observed.*

It is also worth noting that, in a minority of cases, patients experienced adverse effects without any offsetting benefit. Gastrointestinal symptoms, mild liver enzyme elevations, and drug interactions were occasionally reported. These events reinforce the need for **careful monitoring and transparent communication** with healthcare providers, as emphasized throughout this book.

The collective wisdom from these journeys is not one of discouragement, but of **measured realism**. The reported lack of benefit in some cases does not negate the value of inquiry or the importance of patient autonomy. Rather, it illustrates the necessity of approaching any integrative protocol with both curiosity and caution, and of maintaining clear-eyed expectations rooted in the current scientific landscape. Patients and caregivers who shared their experiences often emphasized the importance of ongoing dialogue with medical teams, meticulous record-keeping, and a willingness to reassess strategies as new information emerged.

Ultimately, these stories serve as a reminder that the path through cancer care is rarely linear or predictable. While some may find stabilization or improvement, others will not, despite best efforts and careful adherence. The lessons learned from these less favorable outcomes are invaluable: they foster humility, encourage rigorous evaluation, and reinforce the central role of evidence-based medicine in guiding decisions. For every reported success, there are journeys marked by perseverance in the face of disappointment—a testament to the resilience of patients and families, and a call for continued research and open-minded inquiry in the pursuit of better answers.

10.4 Long-Term Follow-Up & Maintenance

For many patients who have chosen to explore fenbendazole or ivermectin protocols, the initial phase—marked by uncertainty and close observation—gradually gives way to a new set of challenges: the question of how to maintain stability, monitor progress, and adapt over time. Long-term follow-up becomes a dynamic process, shaped both by the unpredictable nature of cancer itself and by the evolving needs of those living with it. Patients and caregivers who have reported positive responses often describe the post-response period not as an endpoint, but as the beginning of a vigilant, ongoing partnership with their own health.

Regular medical follow-up remains the cornerstone of any long-term strategy. Most patients continue to undergo imaging studies, blood tests, and specialist consultations at intervals determined by their oncology teams. These clinical check-ins are essential, not only for detecting recurrence or progression, but also for monitoring organ function—particularly because off-label or non-standard therapies can introduce unknown variables. In practice, patients frequently report bringing detailed logs of their self-administered protocols, including dosages, schedules, and any supplements, to these appointments. This transparency fosters a more collaborative dialogue and allows healthcare professionals to assess potential interactions or cumulative effects.

Adjustments to the protocol are not uncommon. Some individuals, after achieving a period of stability, choose to reduce the frequency or dose of fenbendazole or ivermectin, often in consultation with their physicians or based on their own assessment of side effects and quality of life. Others maintain a steady regimen, guided by the principle of "not fixing what isn't broken," but remain open to change should new symptoms or laboratory findings emerge. Flexibility is a recurring theme: what works for one patient may not be sustainable or optimal for another, and the willingness to adapt—while maintaining rigorous self-observation—proves invaluable.

A number of patients supplement their core protocol with supportive measures aimed at overall well-being and resilience. These can include dietary modifications, targeted nutritional supplements, physical activity adapted to individual capacity, and stress reduction techniques. While the direct impact of these adjuncts on cancer outcomes remains difficult to quantify, many report subjective improvements in energy, mood, and daily functioning. Importantly, these strategies are rarely static; patients often experiment, track results, and refine their approach based on both personal experience and ongoing research.

The psychological dimension of long-term maintenance is significant. Patients describe a heightened sense of vigilance—sometimes bordering on anxiety—around each scan or laboratory result. Over time, however, some develop a more balanced outlook, integrating the protocol into their daily routine without allowing it to dominate their lives. Peer support, whether through online communities or local groups, plays a crucial role in sustaining motivation and providing practical advice. Sharing experiences, setbacks, and small victories helps to normalize the uncertainties inherent in long-term follow-up.

There are also cases where patients, after a sustained period of remission or stable disease, elect to discontinue the protocol altogether. This decision is typically made in close consultation with their medical team and is often accompanied by a plan for intensified surveillance. The rationale can vary: concerns about long-term toxicity, a desire to minimize medication burden, or simply the wish to reclaim a greater sense of normalcy. In these instances, patients emphasize the importance of having clear criteria for re-initiating treatment should new evidence of disease arise.

Throughout these journeys, documentation emerges as a powerful tool. Many patients maintain meticulous records—not only of their protocol and medical results, but also of subjective symptoms, lifestyle changes, and emotional states. Over time, these logs provide a nuanced picture that can inform both personal decision-making and discussions with healthcare providers. In some cases, this level of detail has enabled early detection of subtle changes, prompting timely interventions.

Ultimately, the long-term management of fenbendazole and ivermectin protocols is characterized by **continuous learning and adaptation**. Patients and caregivers who navigate this terrain successfully tend to approach it with a blend of discipline, curiosity, and humility. They recognize the limits of current knowledge, remain alert to new developments in research, and prioritize open communication with their medical teams. While the landscape is still evolving, these experiences underscore the value of a proactive, informed approach—one that balances hope with realism, and innovation with safety.

Chapter 11: The Caregiver's Perspective

11.1 Becoming the Advocate

The role of a caregiver in the context of cancer, particularly when exploring integrative protocols such as those involving fenbendazole and ivermectin, extends well beyond providing comfort and daily assistance. Caregivers often find themselves stepping into the crucial position of advocate—acting as the patient's voice, information manager, and primary liaison with the broader healthcare system. This advocacy is not merely a supportive gesture; it is a complex, dynamic responsibility that can directly influence the quality and continuity of care.

At the heart of effective advocacy lies the ability to synthesize and communicate information. Cancer care today is characterized by an overwhelming volume of data, evolving treatment guidelines, and a proliferation of anecdotal and research-based reports—particularly in the realm of non-traditional protocols. For patients already navigating the physical and emotional toll of their diagnosis, parsing this information can be daunting. The caregiver becomes the *interpreter*, distilling complex medical terminology, weighing the relevance of new studies, and ensuring that nothing essential is overlooked. This often involves maintaining organized records of laboratory results, medication schedules, and notes from consultations, as well as tracking the details of any integrative approaches under consideration.

The advocacy role also demands a proactive stance in communication. Caregivers frequently coordinate between multiple specialists—oncologists, primary care physicians, pharmacists, and, in some cases, practitioners of complementary medicine. Each provider may have a different perspective on the safety, efficacy, and appropriateness of protocols like fenbendazole or ivermectin. The caregiver's task is to facilitate transparent, respectful dialogue, ensuring that the patient's preferences and questions are clearly articulated and that the medical team's responses are understood. This might involve preparing detailed lists of questions before appointments, clarifying points of confusion, or requesting written summaries of recommendations. In situations where language or cultural barriers exist, the caregiver may also act as a cultural broker, helping bridge gaps in understanding and expectation.

Beyond managing information and communication, caregivers often coordinate the logistical aspects of care. This can include scheduling appointments, arranging transportation, managing insurance paperwork, and ensuring that medications—both conventional and integrative—are obtained from reputable sources. In the context of off-label or repurposed drugs, such as those discussed in this book, vigilance is essential. Ensuring the authenticity and safety of medications, verifying dosing regimens, and monitoring for potential interactions or side effects all fall within the caregiver's remit. The ability to anticipate challenges and respond swiftly to emerging issues is a hallmark of effective advocacy.

A particularly nuanced aspect of advocacy involves balancing hope with realism. Patients and families seeking new avenues of treatment are often exposed to a mix of promising anecdotes and sobering scientific realities. The caregiver, as advocate, must help the patient navigate this landscape—encouraging informed optimism while guarding against false hope or unproven claims. This requires a discerning approach to information, a willingness to ask difficult questions, and the emotional resilience to support the patient's choices, even when they diverge from conventional wisdom.

The advocacy journey is rarely linear. It evolves as the patient's condition changes, as new information emerges, and as the emotional landscape shifts. Caregivers who embrace this role with intention and preparation often find that their efforts yield tangible benefits: improved coordination of care, enhanced patient autonomy, and, perhaps most importantly, a sense of shared purpose in the face of uncertainty. The process is demanding, but it is also profoundly meaningful. By becoming the patient's advocate, the caregiver not only supports the logistical and medical aspects of care, but also affirms the patient's dignity, agency, and right to participate fully in decisions about their own health.

Concrete examples illustrate the breadth of this role. Consider the caregiver who maintains a dedicated notebook, documenting every medication change, side effect, and physician comment, and who uses this record to prepare for each clinical visit. Or the spouse who researches the latest studies on fenbendazole, synthesizes the findings, and presents a concise summary to the oncology team, ensuring that the patient's interest in integrative approaches is respected and addressed. In another scenario, an adult child might coordinate a virtual meeting between the patient's oncologist and a complementary medicine specialist, fostering collaboration and reducing the risk of conflicting advice.

Ultimately, effective advocacy is built on a foundation of organization, clear communication, and critical thinking. It requires both attention to detail and the ability to see the bigger picture. For caregivers, these skills are not innate; they are developed over time, often through trial, error, and reflection. The journey is challenging, but the impact is significant—not only for the patient, but for the caregiver themselves, who becomes an indispensable partner in the pursuit of the best possible care.

11.2 Emotional Realities of Supporting a Loved One

The emotional landscape for caregivers supporting a loved one through cancer is often as complex and demanding as the practical responsibilities they shoulder. The daily reality is shaped by a persistent undercurrent of stress, punctuated by moments of acute fear, hope, and—at times—profound exhaustion. While the focus of attention is naturally on the patient, the caregiver's own emotional health is frequently overlooked, despite being a critical component of sustained, effective support.

Caregivers commonly describe a sense of *hypervigilance*—a constant readiness to respond to medical needs, changes in symptoms, or emotional distress. This heightened alertness, while adaptive in the short term, can lead to chronic stress. Physiologically, caregivers may experience disrupted sleep, headaches, or changes in appetite. Psychologically, the pressures can manifest as irritability, anxiety, or a persistent sense of being overwhelmed. The emotional weight is compounded by the unpredictability of the disease course and the ever-present fear of progression or loss.

One of the most challenging aspects is the *dual role* caregivers often assume: providing unwavering support while managing their own emotional responses. Many report feeling that their own grief, anger, or frustration must be suppressed to avoid burdening the patient. This emotional restraint, while well-intentioned, can result in a sense of isolation. For example, a spouse who is the primary caregiver may find herself comforting her partner after a difficult scan, only to retreat to another room to process her own fears in solitude. Over time, this pattern can erode emotional resilience and contribute to burnout.

Resilience, however, is not a fixed trait but a dynamic process. Research in psycho-oncology highlights that caregivers who actively engage in *meaning-making*—finding purpose in their role or connecting caregiving to personal values—tend to experience lower levels of distress. For some, this may involve reframing caregiving as an act of love or service; for others, it is about maintaining a sense of agency in the face of uncertainty. Concrete examples abound: a daughter who creates a daily ritual of journaling to process her emotions, or a partner who joins a support group to share experiences and receive validation from peers.

Effective strategies for self-care are essential, not only for the caregiver's well-being but also for the quality of care they provide. Self-care is often misunderstood as self-indulgence, yet it is, in fact, a *foundational necessity.* Evidence-based approaches include establishing regular routines for sleep, nutrition, and exercise, as well as setting realistic boundaries around caregiving tasks. For instance, scheduling brief periods of respite—whether through the help of family, friends, or professional respite services—can provide much-needed relief. Even small acts, such as taking a daily walk or enjoying a favorite book, can help restore a sense of normalcy and personal identity.

Communication is another pillar of emotional resilience. Caregivers benefit from honest conversations with their loved one about fears, hopes, and limitations. This transparency can reduce misunderstandings and foster a sense of partnership. Equally important is the willingness to seek external support, whether from mental health professionals, spiritual advisors, or peer networks. Many caregivers hesitate to reach out, fearing judgment or the perception of inadequacy. Yet, studies consistently show that those who access support resources report lower levels of depression and anxiety.

Navigating the emotional realities of caregiving also involves recognizing and accepting the limits of one's control. The unpredictability of cancer can trigger a relentless search for answers or solutions, sometimes leading to frustration or guilt when outcomes do not align with effort. It is vital for caregivers to acknowledge that, despite their best intentions and actions, some aspects of the journey are beyond their influence. This acceptance is not resignation but a form of psychological flexibility that allows for adaptation and self-compassion.

The cumulative effect of these emotional challenges and coping strategies shapes the caregiver's experience over time. Some emerge with a renewed sense of purpose and deeper relationships, while others may struggle with lingering grief or exhaustion. The difference often lies in the degree to which caregivers are able to integrate self-care, seek support, and maintain open communication—not only with the patient but also with their own internal experience.

Ultimately, the emotional realities of caregiving are marked by complexity and nuance. Recognizing the legitimacy of one's own feelings, prioritizing self-care, and cultivating resilience are not acts of selfishness but essential elements of sustainable caregiving. In the context of integrative and experimental protocols, such as those explored in earlier chapters, the caregiver's emotional health becomes even more critical—serving as both anchor and compass throughout the uncertainty of the cancer journey.

11.3 Practical Lessons from Caregivers

Experienced caregivers often describe the early days of supporting a loved one through cancer as a rapid immersion into a world of medical appointments, new terminology, and shifting priorities. Over time, their insights coalesce into a set of practical strategies that not only sustain daily care but also preserve the caregiver's own well-being. The most effective approaches are rarely dramatic; rather, they are the result of incremental adjustments—small, deliberate choices that, over weeks and months, create a foundation for resilience.

Organization emerges as a recurring theme in the accounts of seasoned caregivers. The sheer volume of information—medication schedules, lab results, dietary needs, and symptom changes—can quickly become overwhelming. Many caregivers recommend establishing a single, centralized system for tracking this data. Whether using a dedicated notebook, a digital spreadsheet, or a specialized app, the key is consistency and accessibility. For example, one caregiver described maintaining a binder divided into sections: medication logs, appointment calendars, test results, and a running list of questions for the oncology team. This approach not only reduces the risk of errors but also provides a tangible sense of control amidst uncertainty. Others have found value in color-coding pill organizers or setting phone alarms for medication times, transforming complex regimens into manageable routines.

Communication, both within the family and with the healthcare team, requires ongoing attention and skill. Caregivers frequently serve as the primary liaison between the patient and multiple specialists, translating medical jargon and ensuring that everyone remains informed. One practical lesson is to prepare for each medical visit by reviewing recent symptoms, documenting any side effects, and writing down specific questions. This preparation enables more focused, efficient consultations and helps prevent important concerns from being overlooked. Additionally, experienced caregivers emphasize the value of honest, open dialogue at home. Regular family check-ins, even brief ones, can surface unspoken worries and clarify expectations, reducing misunderstandings and emotional strain. Some families have adopted shared digital calendars or messaging groups to coordinate visits, meals, and errands, ensuring that support is distributed and no single person becomes overwhelmed.

Managing the day-to-day realities of care often means balancing structure with flexibility. Rigid routines can quickly unravel in the face of unexpected test results or sudden changes in the patient's condition. Seasoned caregivers advise building routines around anchor points—such as mealtimes, medication windows, or daily walks—while allowing for adjustments as needed. This approach creates a rhythm that supports both patient and caregiver, while acknowledging that unpredictability is part of the landscape. For instance, one caregiver described how she and her partner developed a "morning review," a brief conversation to assess the patient's energy and symptoms, which then informed the plan for the day. This practice fostered a sense of partnership and adaptability, rather than frustration when plans inevitably changed.

Self-care is not a luxury but a necessity, as many caregivers learn through experience. The demands of caregiving can erode physical and emotional reserves, making it essential to schedule regular breaks and accept help when offered. Some caregivers have found it helpful to create a rotating list of friends or family members who can provide respite, even for short periods. Others have built restorative practices into their own routines—short walks, meditation, or simply a quiet cup of tea. These moments of pause are not signs of weakness, but investments in the caregiver's capacity to sustain support over the long term.

Finally, experienced caregivers consistently highlight the importance of documentation—not only for medical and logistical purposes, but as a tool for reflection and advocacy. Keeping a brief daily journal of symptoms, mood changes, and significant events can reveal patterns that might otherwise go unnoticed. This record becomes invaluable when discussing treatment responses or side effects with the healthcare team, and it can also serve as a source of reassurance during difficult periods, providing evidence of progress or stability.

In sum, the practical lessons distilled from caregivers' experiences reflect a blend of structure and adaptability, clear communication, and a commitment to self-preservation. These strategies do not eliminate the challenges of caregiving, but they do offer a roadmap for navigating them with greater confidence and clarity. By sharing these insights, caregivers not only support their loved ones more effectively but also contribute to a culture of informed, compassionate care.

PART VI
TOOLS & CHECKLISTS

CHAPTER 12: STEP-BY-STEP PLANNING TOOLS

12.1 TREATMENT PLANNING CHECKLIST

Effective treatment planning is a cornerstone of any integrative approach to cancer care, particularly when considering protocols that fall outside standard medical pathways. A robust, well-structured checklist not only clarifies the path ahead but also empowers patients and caregivers to engage actively and knowledgeably with their healthcare teams. The following framework is designed to guide readers through the essential steps of planning, implementing, and monitoring a treatment protocol involving fenbendazole, ivermectin, or related supportive measures.

The first step is to define clear, realistic objectives. This means articulating what you hope to achieve—whether it's tumor stabilization, symptom relief, improved quality of life, or a specific biomarker response. These goals should be discussed openly with your medical team, ensuring they align with your overall care plan and personal values. For example, a patient with advanced colorectal cancer might prioritize maintaining energy and independence, while another may focus on maximizing time with family. **Clarity of purpose** is essential, as it shapes every subsequent decision.

Once objectives are established, the next phase involves selecting the therapies to be included in your protocol. This requires careful consideration of the available evidence, personal health status, and compatibility with ongoing conventional treatments. For instance, some patients may choose to integrate fenbendazole based on emerging preclinical data and anecdotal reports, while others might opt for ivermectin due to its distinct mechanisms and safety profile. It is critical to document the exact formulations, dosages, and schedules under consideration. This documentation not only aids memory but also facilitates transparent communication with your healthcare providers.

Equally important is a candid assessment of available resources. This encompasses not only the medications themselves but also supportive supplements, access to laboratory monitoring, and logistical factors such as transportation and financial considerations. For example, a patient living in a rural area may need to coordinate with local pharmacies or consider reliable online sources, always verifying authenticity and quality. **Resource mapping** should extend to supportive care—nutritional counseling, psychological support, and the involvement of family or friends in daily routines.

With therapies and resources defined, constructing a detailed calendar becomes the operational backbone of the plan. This calendar should outline start dates, dosing intervals, anticipated check-ins with the medical team, and scheduled laboratory or imaging assessments. For example, a typical cycle might involve daily fenbendazole administration for three weeks, followed by a rest period, with bloodwork scheduled at baseline and after each cycle. Integrating reminders for symptom tracking and medication adherence can be invaluable, especially when protocols become complex.

Monitoring progress is a dynamic, ongoing process. It involves systematic tracking of both objective measures—such as imaging results, tumor markers, and laboratory values—and subjective experiences, including side effects, energy levels, sleep quality, and mood. Many patients find it helpful to maintain a dedicated treatment journal or use digital tools to log daily observations. This record becomes a powerful asset during consultations, enabling more precise adjustments and fostering shared decision-making.

Throughout this process, regular communication with the healthcare team remains paramount. Bringing a concise, well-organized summary of your protocol—including objectives, therapies, schedules, and observed effects—to each appointment ensures that your care remains coordinated and safe. It also signals to clinicians that you are approaching complementary therapies with seriousness and discernment, which can foster a more collaborative relationship.

Consider the example of a caregiver supporting a loved one through a complex protocol. By maintaining a shared document that tracks medication administration, side effects, and questions for the next medical visit, the caregiver not only reduces the risk of errors but also alleviates some of the emotional burden associated with uncertainty. This structured approach can transform a daunting process into a manageable, even empowering, experience.

Ultimately, a comprehensive treatment planning checklist serves not just as an organizational tool, but as a blueprint for active participation in care. It bridges the gap between emerging scientific insights and the lived realities of patients and families. By systematically addressing objectives, therapies, resources, scheduling, and monitoring, individuals can navigate the complexities of integrative protocols with greater confidence and clarity—always anchored by the understanding that these efforts are most effective when pursued in close partnership with the broader medical team.

12.2 Questions for Your Doctor or Care Team

The process of integrating any new treatment—especially those outside standard protocols—requires careful, informed dialogue with your healthcare team. Systematic verification through targeted questions is essential to ensure that all relevant aspects are considered, potential risks are understood, and expectations are aligned. This checklist is designed to help you approach these conversations with clarity and confidence, ensuring that no critical issue is overlooked and that your decisions are grounded in both scientific evidence and your unique clinical context.

A well-structured set of questions serves several purposes. It not only clarifies the scientific rationale and safety profile of reported protocols but also helps you and your care team identify potential interactions, contraindications, and monitoring strategies. By preparing in advance, you create space for a more open, productive dialogue—one that supports shared decision-making and respects both medical expertise and your lived experience.

Essential Questions for Your Doctor or Care Team: Verification Checklist

These items help ensure comprehensive coverage and quality control:

- **What are the potential risks and side effects of fenbendazole or ivermectin in my specific situation?**

Understanding the unique risk profile is critical, as individual factors such as comorbidities, current medications, and cancer type can influence safety.

Ask for details on known adverse effects, rare complications, and any patient-specific considerations.

- **What are the potential benefits, and what does current research suggest about effectiveness for my cancer type?**

It is important to distinguish between anecdotal reports and evidence-based outcomes.

Request a summary of the latest research, including any limitations or uncertainties, and how these may relate to your case.

- **Are there any known interactions with my current treatments or medications?**

Drug-drug interactions can alter efficacy or increase toxicity.

Provide a complete list of your medications and supplements, and ask if any combinations are contraindicated.

- What alternative or complementary options should I consider?

Exploring all available choices ensures a balanced perspective and may reveal safer or more effective strategies.

Discuss both conventional and integrative therapies relevant to your diagnosis and goals.

- How will we monitor for efficacy and side effects if I proceed with this protocol?

Ongoing assessment is essential for early identification of complications or lack of benefit.

Clarify what tests, symptoms, or biomarkers will be tracked, and how frequently monitoring will occur.

- What are realistic expectations regarding outcomes, both short- and long-term?

Setting clear expectations helps prevent disappointment and supports informed consent.

Ask about possible timelines for response, likelihood of benefit, and signs that may prompt discontinuation.

- What is the recommended dosing, schedule, and duration for this protocol in my context?

Accurate dosing is crucial for both safety and potential efficacy.

Request specific guidance tailored to your weight, organ function, and treatment history.

- Who will coordinate and oversee this aspect of my care?

Clear roles reduce confusion and ensure accountability.

Identify which member of your team will monitor progress, handle questions, and adjust the protocol if needed.

- What should I do if I experience new or worsening symptoms?

Prompt reporting of adverse events can prevent serious complications.

Establish clear instructions for when and how to contact your team, and what symptoms require urgent attention.

- Are there any legal, regulatory, or supply considerations I should be aware of?

Some medications may not be approved for human use or may have supply chain issues.

Discuss the legal status, sourcing, and any documentation required for off-label or veterinary drugs.

Using This Checklist:

- Bring this checklist to appointments as a reference; use it to guide your conversation and take notes on your team's responses.
- Not every item will apply to every situation—adapt questions based on your diagnosis, treatment history, and personal priorities.
- If time is limited, prioritize the questions most relevant to your immediate concerns and follow up as needed.

Quality Assurance:

- Review your notes after the discussion to confirm that all key points were addressed.
- If any answers are unclear or incomplete, request clarification or a follow-up appointment.
- Successful verification means you understand the rationale, risks, and monitoring plan for any protocol under consideration, and feel confident in your next steps.

A systematic approach to questioning not only empowers you as a participant in your care but also fosters a collaborative relationship with your healthcare team. By ensuring that each of these areas is addressed, you reduce uncertainty, enhance safety, and support the best possible outcomes—no matter where your treatment journey leads.

CHAPTER 13: QUICK REFERENCE GUIDE

13.1 KEY SAFETY POINTS (DO'S & DON'TS)

In any context where off-label or repurposed medications are being considered—especially in oncology—systematic safety verification is not just prudent, but essential. The reported use of fenbendazole and ivermectin by patients navigating complex cancer journeys introduces unique variables and potential risks. A structured approach ensures that critical details are not missed, and that decision-making remains grounded in evidence, vigilance, and open communication with healthcare professionals.

This checklist distills the essential do's and don'ts for anyone considering or actively using these protocols. It is designed to help patients and caregivers proactively identify potential hazards, optimize monitoring, and maintain the highest standards of safety. Each item is accompanied by a brief rationale, clarifying its importance and offering practical guidance on what to verify. The goal is to support informed, confident participation in care, while minimizing avoidable complications.

Safety Verification Checklist: Essential Do's & Don'ts for Reported Fenbendazole and Ivermectin Use

- **Consultation with Oncology Team Before Initiation**

Direct communication with your oncologist or primary cancer care provider is non-negotiable. This ensures that any protocol is evaluated in the context of your specific diagnosis, treatment plan, and medical history.

Verify that your healthcare team is aware of your intent, and document their guidance or concerns.

- **Verification of Product Authenticity and Purity**

Medications sourced outside of standard pharmaceutical channels may carry risks of contamination, incorrect dosing, or counterfeit ingredients.

Confirm the source, batch number, and, if possible, request a certificate of analysis or independent verification of product quality.

- **Baseline Laboratory Assessment**

Establishing baseline liver and kidney function, complete blood count, and other relevant labs is critical before starting any new agent with systemic effects.

Review recent laboratory results with your physician and ensure that any abnormalities are addressed prior to initiation.

- Drug Interaction Screening

Fenbendazole and ivermectin can interact with conventional cancer therapies, supportive medications, or supplements, potentially altering efficacy or safety.

Request a thorough drug interaction check from your pharmacist or oncologist, with particular attention to chemotherapy, immunotherapy, anticoagulants, and anticonvulsants.

- Clear Understanding of Dosing Protocols

Reported regimens vary widely, and dosing errors can lead to toxicity or subtherapeutic exposure.

Confirm the intended dose, frequency, and duration based on the most credible sources available; avoid arbitrary adjustments without medical input.

- Monitoring for Adverse Effects

Both medications have documented side effects, some of which may overlap with symptoms of cancer or its treatments.

Maintain a symptom diary, noting any new or worsening issues such as gastrointestinal disturbances, neurological symptoms, allergic reactions, or changes in laboratory values.

- Prompt Reporting of Concerning Symptoms

Early identification of adverse reactions can prevent escalation to severe toxicity.

Establish clear criteria for when to contact your healthcare team – such as persistent vomiting, jaundice, confusion, severe rash, or unexplained fever.

- Avoidance of Simultaneous Initiation with New Therapies

Starting multiple new agents at once complicates attribution of side effects and increases risk.

Introduce one protocol at a time, with a defined observation period before adding or changing other therapies.

- Documentation of All Substances Taken

A comprehensive, up-to-date medication and supplement list supports safer care and more accurate medical decision-making.

Record all prescription drugs, over-the-counter medications, supplements, and any non-conventional agents being used.

- **Respect for Regulatory and Legal Considerations**

The use of veterinary or non-approved formulations in humans may have legal and regulatory implications, depending on jurisdiction.

Familiarize yourself with local laws and discuss any concerns with your healthcare provider.

USING THIS CHECKLIST:

- Refer to this checklist before starting, and periodically during, any reported protocol involving fenbendazole or ivermectin.
- Tailor the checklist to your individual situation—some items may not apply in every case, but all represent best-practice considerations.
- If uncertainty arises or a checklist item cannot be verified, pause and seek clarification from a qualified healthcare professional before proceeding.

QUALITY ASSURANCE:

- Thoroughly review each item, ideally in collaboration with your healthcare team, to ensure no critical steps are overlooked.
- Successful verification means each box is checked with confidence, supported by documentation or direct communication with medical professionals.

A systematic approach to safety is a cornerstone of responsible, patient-centered care—especially when exploring integrative or complementary options. By methodically verifying each aspect of protocol use, patients and caregivers can reduce uncertainty, prevent avoidable harm, and engage more effectively with their healthcare teams. This checklist is not merely a formality, but a practical safeguard—one that empowers you to navigate complex decisions with clarity and confidence.

13.2 Resource Links (Research Hubs & Patient Communities)

Navigating the landscape of research and community support is essential for anyone considering integrative approaches such as fenbendazole and ivermectin. The digital era has brought a wealth of resources, but also a challenge: distinguishing credible, up-to-date information from speculation or misinformation. The following curated list represents the most reliable online hubs, clinical registries, and patient communities relevant to these protocols. Each resource is selected for its professional standing, active oversight, and practical utility for patients and caregivers.

ClinicalTrials.gov stands as the gold standard for tracking ongoing and completed clinical research worldwide. Maintained by the U.S. National Library of Medicine, this database allows users to search for studies involving fenbendazole, ivermectin, or related compounds. It provides detailed study protocols, eligibility criteria, and—when available—results and published findings. For patients and caregivers seeking to understand the current research landscape or to identify potential trial participation opportunities, this registry is indispensable.

PubMed, also managed by the National Library of Medicine, is the premier repository for peer-reviewed biomedical literature. A targeted search for "fenbendazole cancer," "ivermectin oncology," or similar terms yields a curated list of scientific articles, reviews, and case reports. PubMed's advanced filters enable users to focus on recent publications, clinical trials, or systematic reviews, offering a reliable foundation for evidence-based decision-making. For those wishing to delve deeper into the science, PubMed remains the definitive starting point.

The National Cancer Institute (NCI) provides a robust suite of resources, including research summaries, drug information, and patient guides. While fenbendazole and ivermectin are not standard components of NCI-endorsed cancer regimens, the Institute's website offers authoritative background on cancer biology, investigational therapies, and patient advocacy. The NCI's Cancer Information Service also offers personalized support via phone or live chat, helping users interpret research findings and connect with clinical experts.

For those interested in the European research context, the European Clinical Trials Register offers a comprehensive database of studies conducted within the European Union and European Economic Area. This platform mirrors the transparency and rigor of ClinicalTrials.gov, and can be particularly valuable for patients seeking trials or research updates outside the United States. Its multilingual interface and detailed trial records support informed engagement with the evolving field of integrative oncology.

Beyond research hubs, patient communities play a vital role in sharing practical insights, lived experiences, and emotional support. Inspire's Cancer Support Community, for example, hosts moderated forums where patients and caregivers discuss a wide range of treatments, including off-label and experimental protocols. While anecdotal, these discussions often reveal real-world challenges, coping strategies, and questions to bring to one's medical team. The community's moderation and partnership with established cancer organizations help maintain a constructive, respectful environment.

Reddit's r/cancer and r/AskDocs subreddits, though informal, have become gathering places for patients exploring unconventional therapies. These forums allow for candid discussion, peer-to-peer advice, and rapid sharing of new research or media reports. It is crucial, however, to approach such platforms with discernment: while they can surface valuable questions and highlight emerging trends, medical advice should always be validated through professional channels.

The Anticancer Fund, a non-profit organization based in Belgium, is recognized for its commitment to evidence-based information on repurposed drugs in oncology. Its website features detailed drug profiles, research updates, and patient guides that critically appraise the state of the science for agents like ivermectin and fenbendazole. The Fund's focus on transparency and patient empowerment aligns closely with the ethos of this handbook.

Finally, Smart Patients offers a unique blend of expert moderation and patient-driven dialogue. Its cancer forums include discussions on integrative and experimental treatments, with an emphasis on respectful, informed exchange. Members often share personal protocols, supplement regimens, and experiences with healthcare teams, providing a nuanced perspective that bridges the gap between research and daily practice.

In summary, these resources collectively empower patients and caregivers to move beyond isolated anecdotes and unverified claims. By combining the rigor of clinical registries and scientific databases with the lived wisdom of patient communities, readers are equipped to ask sharper questions, monitor developments, and engage proactively with their healthcare teams. As the field of integrative oncology evolves, these hubs will remain essential waypoints for anyone seeking clarity, connection, and credible guidance.

CHAPTER 14: CONCLUSION – CRITICAL OUTLOOK & FUTURE DIRECTIONS

14.1 STRENGTH OF CURRENT EVIDENCE

The evidence base for fenbendazole and ivermectin in oncology is a landscape defined by promise, complexity, and significant gaps. A critical appraisal requires distinguishing among three distinct strata: preclinical data, clinical research, and anecdotal or patient-reported experiences. Each layer contributes uniquely to our understanding, but also carries inherent limitations that must be acknowledged with precision.

Preclinical studies—those conducted in vitro (cell cultures) or in vivo (animal models)—form the foundation of scientific interest in both fenbendazole and ivermectin as potential anticancer agents. Fenbendazole, originally developed as an anthelmintic for veterinary use, has demonstrated the ability to disrupt microtubule dynamics in cancer cells, inhibit glucose uptake, and induce apoptosis across several tumor cell lines. Ivermectin, similarly, has shown cytotoxicity against a range of cancer types, with mechanisms involving modulation of the Wnt/β-catenin pathway, inhibition of multidrug resistance proteins, and interference with cellular signaling essential for tumor survival. These findings are robust within the controlled environment of the laboratory, where concentrations, exposure times, and biological contexts are carefully managed. Such studies provide compelling mechanistic rationale and have fueled the hypothesis that these agents might offer benefit beyond their original indications.

However, the leap from preclinical promise to clinical reality is substantial. The translation of laboratory results into meaningful outcomes for human patients is fraught with challenges. Differences in drug metabolism, tumor microenvironment, immune system interactions, and the complexity of human disease often render preclinical successes only partially predictive of clinical efficacy. In the case of fenbendazole, there are currently no published, peer-reviewed clinical trials that systematically evaluate its safety or effectiveness in cancer patients. The clinical literature on ivermectin is somewhat broader, primarily due to its established use in humans for parasitic infections. A handful of early-phase trials and case reports have explored its anticancer potential, particularly in hematologic malignancies and some solid tumors, but these studies are preliminary. They are often limited by small sample sizes, lack of control groups, and short follow-up periods. As a result, the clinical evidence remains **insufficient to support routine use** of either agent in oncology outside of research settings.

Anecdotal reports and patient-driven protocols, widely circulated on online forums and social media, have played a significant role in shaping public perception. Stories of individuals experiencing remission or disease stabilization after incorporating fenbendazole or ivermectin into their regimen are undeniably compelling. These narratives often reflect the desperation and resourcefulness of patients facing advanced disease with limited options. While such accounts can offer valuable insights into real-world experiences, they are inherently subject to bias, placebo effects, and confounding factors. Without systematic data collection, standardized dosing, or objective outcome measures, it is impossible to determine causality or generalize these results to broader patient populations. The risk of overestimating benefit—or underestimating harm—based on anecdotal evidence is substantial.

It is also essential to recognize the role of *publication bias* and the tendency for positive outcomes to be shared more widely than negative or neutral experiences. In the absence of rigorous clinical trials, the true risk-benefit profile of these agents in oncology remains undefined. This uncertainty underscores the importance of critical appraisal and the need for patients and caregivers to maintain open, evidence-informed dialogue with their healthcare teams.

Despite these limitations, the scientific community has taken notice. The mechanistic plausibility demonstrated in preclinical work has prompted calls for well-designed clinical trials. Regulatory agencies and academic institutions are increasingly aware of the demand for alternative and adjunctive therapies, particularly for patients with refractory cancers. Until such trials are completed and published, however, the strength of current evidence must be regarded as *suggestive but not conclusive*. The prudent approach is to view fenbendazole and ivermectin as investigational agents in oncology—worthy of further study, but not yet validated for routine clinical use.

In summary, the current evidence supporting the use of fenbendazole and ivermectin in cancer care is strongest at the preclinical level, with intriguing laboratory data but a notable absence of high-quality clinical research. Anecdotal experiences, while meaningful on a personal level, cannot substitute for systematic investigation. For patients and caregivers, this means navigating a landscape of hope, uncertainty, and the ongoing need for critical engagement with emerging data. The future may hold more definitive answers, but at present, careful scrutiny and informed skepticism remain essential.

14.2 Limitations and Research Gaps

Despite the growing interest in fenbendazole and ivermectin as potential adjuncts in cancer care, the current body of evidence is marked by significant limitations and research gaps that must be acknowledged with clarity and precision. These limitations are not merely academic; they have direct implications for patients and caregivers seeking to make informed, responsible decisions.

The most evident constraint is the **lack of large-scale, randomized controlled trials (RCTs)** evaluating the efficacy and safety of fenbendazole and ivermectin in human oncology. Much of the enthusiasm surrounding these agents stems from *preclinical studies*—in vitro experiments and animal models—that, while promising, cannot reliably predict clinical outcomes in humans. The leap from laboratory findings to therapeutic protocols is substantial, and without robust clinical trials, any conclusions about effectiveness remain speculative. For example, while fenbendazole has demonstrated anti-tumor activity in various cell lines and animal studies, these results have not yet been substantiated by peer-reviewed human trials with rigorous methodology.

Another significant limitation lies in the **heterogeneity of reported patient experiences**. Anecdotal accounts and case reports, although valuable for hypothesis generation, are inherently subject to bias, confounding factors, and placebo effects. These narratives often lack standardized dosing regimens, consistent monitoring, or objective outcome measures. Consequently, it becomes difficult to discern whether observed improvements are attributable to the intervention, concurrent therapies, natural disease fluctuations, or other variables. This variability underscores the need for systematic data collection and standardized reporting protocols.

The **pharmacokinetics and pharmacodynamics** of both fenbendazole and ivermectin in cancer patients remain poorly characterized. Most available data pertain to their use in veterinary or antiparasitic contexts, not oncology. Factors such as absorption, metabolism, tissue distribution, and potential interactions with chemotherapeutic agents are insufficiently understood. For patients already navigating complex treatment regimens, these unknowns introduce additional risks. There is also a paucity of information regarding optimal dosing schedules, duration of therapy, and potential cumulative toxicities when these agents are used over extended periods or in combination with other drugs.

A further research gap exists in the **identification of patient subgroups who might benefit—or be harmed—by these interventions**. Cancer is not a monolithic disease; genetic, molecular, and immunological profiles vary widely between individuals and tumor types. The absence of biomarker-driven studies or stratified analyses means that any observed effects may not be generalizable. For instance, certain mutations or tumor microenvironment characteristics could theoretically influence responsiveness to microtubule inhibitors like fenbendazole, yet these nuances remain largely unexplored.

Safety data, particularly regarding long-term use and rare adverse events, are notably limited. While both drugs have established safety profiles in their approved indications, off-label use in oncology—often at different doses or durations—raises new questions. Reports of hepatotoxicity, neurotoxicity, and hypersensitivity reactions, though rare, warrant systematic investigation. The risk of drug-drug interactions, especially in polypharmacy scenarios common among cancer patients, is another area where empirical data are lacking.

Additionally, there is a **deficit of research addressing the psychological and social dimensions** of self-directed or adjunctive therapy with these agents. The decision to pursue non-standard treatments is often made in the context of hope, uncertainty, and sometimes desperation. Understanding the impact of these choices on patient quality of life, emotional well-being, and the doctor-patient relationship is as important as elucidating biological mechanisms.

Finally, regulatory and ethical considerations present their own set of challenges. The absence of clear guidelines for off-label use, coupled with the proliferation of unverified information online, can leave patients vulnerable to misinformation or exploitation. There is a pressing need for frameworks that balance innovation with patient safety, ensuring that new avenues are explored responsibly and transparently.

In summary, while the scientific rationale for investigating fenbendazole and ivermectin in oncology is compelling, the current landscape is defined by **gaps in clinical evidence, pharmacological understanding, safety data, and ethical guidance**. Addressing these limitations requires coordinated efforts: well-designed clinical trials, rigorous pharmacological studies, transparent reporting of both positive and negative outcomes, and a commitment to patient-centered research. Only through such comprehensive inquiry can the true potential—and the boundaries—of these protocols be responsibly defined.

14.3 Where the Pipeline Is Heading

The research pipeline for fenbendazole and ivermectin in oncology is entering a pivotal phase, shaped by both the momentum of patient-driven interest and the increasing attention of the scientific community. While early investigations have been largely preclinical or anecdotal, the landscape is evolving as more rigorous studies are initiated and as regulatory bodies begin to acknowledge the need for systematic evaluation. This transition is not merely procedural; it reflects a broader shift in oncology research, where repurposing established drugs for new indications—especially those outside their original scope—has become a strategic priority.

One of the most promising developments is the emergence of well-structured clinical trials designed to address the fundamental questions that preclinical data and patient reports have raised. Several academic centers and independent research groups are now moving beyond cell cultures and animal models to test fenbendazole and ivermectin in controlled human studies. These trials are focusing on various cancer types, dosing regimens, and combination strategies, often in patients with limited options after standard therapies. The design of these studies increasingly incorporates biomarkers and molecular profiling, which may help identify subgroups of patients more likely to benefit from such interventions. This personalized approach is a marked departure from the one-size-fits-all protocols of the past and could be transformative in determining the real-world utility of these agents.

Parallel to formal clinical trials, there is a growing emphasis on *real-world evidence*—systematic collection of data from patients who are already using these protocols outside of research settings. Digital health platforms, patient registries, and collaborative networks are enabling the aggregation of outcomes, side effects, and quality-of-life measures at an unprecedented scale. This data, while not a substitute for randomized trials, can provide valuable signals about safety and efficacy, especially in rare cancers or unique patient populations that may not be well represented in traditional studies. The integration of such *real-world* insights with formal research could accelerate the identification of promising uses and highlight areas where caution is warranted.

Innovation is also being driven by advances in drug delivery and formulation. Researchers are exploring ways to enhance the bioavailability and tumor-targeting properties of fenbendazole and ivermectin, addressing some of the pharmacokinetic limitations observed in earlier studies. Nanoparticle carriers, liposomal formulations, and prodrug strategies are under investigation, with the aim of maximizing therapeutic concentrations at the tumor site while minimizing systemic toxicity. These technological advances could significantly expand the therapeutic window and enable more precise dosing, particularly in combination with other anticancer agents.

Another area of active exploration is the synergy between repurposed antiparasitic agents and established cancer treatments. Preclinical studies suggest that fenbendazole and ivermectin may sensitize tumor cells to chemotherapy, radiation, or immunotherapy by disrupting key cellular pathways. Some ongoing trials are explicitly designed to test these combinations, with the hope of enhancing response rates or overcoming resistance in refractory cancers. If these synergistic effects are confirmed in clinical settings, they could redefine the role of these agents—not as standalone therapies, but as integral components of *multimodal* treatment strategies.

The regulatory environment is also adapting, albeit cautiously. Agencies such as the FDA and EMA are increasingly receptive to drug repurposing initiatives, especially when there is a compelling scientific rationale and unmet clinical need. Accelerated approval pathways, orphan drug designations, and adaptive trial designs are being leveraged to facilitate the evaluation of non-traditional agents in oncology. However, the bar for safety and efficacy remains high, and robust evidence will be required before these protocols can transition from experimental to mainstream care.

Looking ahead, the impact of ongoing and future studies will extend beyond the direct use of fenbendazole and ivermectin. Their investigation is catalyzing broader discussions about patient autonomy, the integration of patient-reported outcomes into research, and the democratization of clinical trial participation. It is also prompting a reevaluation of how anecdotal evidence and grassroots innovation can inform formal scientific inquiry, without compromising rigor or patient safety.

In summary, the research pipeline for fenbendazole and ivermectin is characterized by cautious optimism and a commitment to evidence-based progress. The coming years will likely see a convergence of clinical trial data, real-world evidence, and technological innovation, each informing and reinforcing the other. The ultimate impact will depend not only on the outcomes of these studies, but also on the ability of the medical community to translate findings into safe, effective, and accessible treatment options. For patients and caregivers navigating complex decisions, these developments represent both hope and a reminder of the importance of critical engagement with emerging science.

14.4 WHAT THE MEDICAL COMMUNITY SAYS

Within the medical community, the discussion surrounding the off-label use of fenbendazole and ivermectin in oncology is marked by both caution and curiosity. The prevailing stance among oncologists and scientific societies is one of *measured skepticism*, grounded in the principles of evidence-based medicine. Major organizations such as the American Society of Clinical Oncology (ASCO) and the European Society for Medical Oncology (ESMO) consistently emphasize the necessity of robust clinical trials before endorsing any new therapeutic approach, particularly those repurposing drugs from veterinary or antiparasitic origins. Their official statements, while not dismissive of the underlying scientific rationale, underscore the absence of large-scale, peer-reviewed clinical data supporting efficacy or safety in humans with cancer.

Expert opinion within academic and clinical oncology tends to align with this cautious approach. Leading voices in the field often acknowledge the intriguing preclinical data—laboratory studies and animal models demonstrating anti-tumor effects of both fenbendazole and ivermectin. However, they point out that *translating these findings into meaningful clinical benefit for patients is a complex, multi-step process*. The leap from cell culture or animal studies to human application is fraught with challenges, including differences in metabolism, dosing, and potential for unforeseen toxicity. As a result, most experts refrain from recommending these agents outside of well-designed clinical trials, and many actively discourage self-administration due to the risk of adverse effects, drug interactions, and the potential for undermining established treatments.

Despite this prevailing conservatism, there are pockets of the medical community—often at the intersection of integrative and translational oncology—where interest in drug repurposing is more pronounced. Some clinicians, particularly those involved in early-phase research or compassionate use programs, express a willingness to consider off-label options for patients with advanced, refractory disease. In these contexts, the decision is typically made on a case-by-case basis, with full transparency regarding the experimental nature of the approach and a strong emphasis on informed consent. Even here, the consensus is that such interventions should be closely monitored and ideally conducted within the framework of a clinical study or registry.

It is important to note that the debate is not purely academic. Patient advocacy groups and some individual practitioners have called for accelerated access to promising repurposed drugs, citing the urgent needs of those with limited options. This has, at times, led to tension between patient-driven demand and the cautious pace of regulatory and scientific validation. Some experts warn that anecdotal reports and social media-driven narratives can create unrealistic expectations, potentially exposing vulnerable patients to harm or disappointment. Others, however, argue that the history of oncology is replete with examples of breakthroughs arising from unexpected sources, and that the medical community should remain open to rigorous investigation of novel hypotheses, even those originating outside traditional pharmaceutical pipelines.

The divergence of views within the medical community reflects broader philosophical questions about innovation, risk, and patient autonomy. While the majority of oncologists and scientific bodies advocate for a methodical, data-driven approach, a minority—often motivated by compassion for those facing dire prognoses—are willing to explore unconventional options under carefully controlled circumstances. Ultimately, the consensus remains that patient safety and scientific rigor must guide all decisions, and that any potential role for fenbendazole or ivermectin in cancer care will depend on the outcomes of ongoing and future research.

In practical terms, this means that patients and caregivers considering these protocols should expect their healthcare providers to express caution, request evidence, and prioritize established standards of care. Open, respectful dialogue is essential, as is the recognition that the landscape may evolve with new data. For now, the medical community's position is clear: hope must be balanced by evidence, and innovation must proceed hand in hand with patient protection.

Made in the USA
Coppell, TX
12 October 2025

55084709R00066